S... Hospital Reform

State Hospital Reform

Why Was It So Hard to Accomplish?

Edited by
David B. Pharis

CAROLINA ACADEMIC PRESS
Durham, North Carolina

Copyright © 1998
David B. Pharis
All Rights Reserved

Library of Congress Cataloging-in-Publication Data

State hospital reform : why was it so hard to accomplish? / edited by
David B. Pharis.
    p.   cm.
    Includes bibliographical references (p.).
    ISBN 0-89089-886-3
    1. State hospitals—Texas—History. 2. Psychiatric hospital
patients—Abuse of—Texas. 3. Mental health services—Texas.
4. Texas. Dept. of Mental Health and Mental Retardation—Trial,
litigation, etc. I. Pharis, David B. (David Bunsen), 1941– .
RC445.T37S82   1998
362.2'1'09764—dc21   98-40711
                                              CIP

CAROLINA ACADEMIC PRESS
700 Kent Street
Durham, North Carolina 27701
Telephone (919) 489-7486
Fax (919) 493-5668
E-mail: cap@cap-press.com
www.cap-press.com

Printed in the United States of America.

*For the patients and staff of
Texas's eight state psychiatric hospitals*

Contents

Foreword
David Mechanic   ix

Acknowledgments   xiii

Chapter 1   Reminiscences
David Bell, Patsy Cheyney, Mary Dees,
Susan Medlin, and Anonymous   3

Chapter 2   May Our Tears Be Turned Into Dancing
Genevieve Tarlton Hearon   25

Chapter 3   History of Mental Health Legal Issues
David B. Pharis   53

Chapter 4   The History of the R.A.J. Lawsuit in Texas
David B. Pharis   63

Chapter 5   Reform through Litigation:
A Commissioner's Perspective
Gary E. Miller   99

Chapter 6   The Positive Impact of R.A.J.
Don Gilbert   123

Chapter 7   Measurement of Psychiatric Care
David B. Pharis and Douglas Heinrichs   141

Chapter 8   The Excursion into the Community
David B. Pharis   159

Chapter 9   Evaluating Compliance with the
Aftercare Standards
Howard H. Goldman and
Anne Mathews Younes   181

Chapter 10   Politics and Costs
David B. Pharis   193

Contents

Chapter 11	Quality System Oversight *David Axelrad*	217
Chapter 12	The Consultants' Assessment of the Quality System Oversight Process *Arthur J. Farley, E. R. Hayes, Marty Lumpkin, Charles McDonald, Marilyn Clark, Lyn Henderson, Felicia Korman, Cynthia Patton Duran, William Smith, and Hazel Byers*	253
Chapter 13	The Legacy of R.A.J. from the Court's Perspective *Barefoot Sanders*	273
Afterword	*David Mechanic*	279
Contributors		283

Foreword

David Mechanic

In the 1960's and 1970's, public interest attorneys, fresh from impressive victories in the civil rights arena, turned their attention to care for persons with mental illness. Those were heady days with great optimism that the courts could be used as instruments for social changes that legislatures and executives were unwilling to advance. With some precedents in California and Washington, D.C., Charles Halperin and his colleagues, at the Center for Law and Social Policy, brought a class action suit in Alabama in 1970, Wyatt v. Stickney, maintaining a constitutional right to treatment. Having found a sympathetic and activist U.S. District Court judge (Frank Johnson), the litigators took Alabama on a trajectory of requirements that was to change its mental health system and have reverberations throughout the nation.

The mental health bar sought constitutional and other bases to define a right to treatment, to restrain civil commitment procedures and introduce substantial due process, and to develop a right to refuse treatment. Lawyers developed novel legal theories that would allow them to extend protections for involuntary hospitalization to care in the community which was becoming the major locus of patient management. Looking back, in Paul Appelbaum's phrase it was "Almost a Revolution," but one that had more limits than enthusiasts once believed. Even then it should have been apparent that having courts substitute for legislative and professional decisions about how to best use limited health resources, however well intentioned, could result in unanticipated and perverse consequences. Political changes and public opinion eventually tempered judicial mental health activism but the courts also pulled back as judges began to appreciate more deeply some of the difficulties and dilemmas involved in care and treatment and the best use of public resources.

Early court decisions that set standards of care often resulted in wholesale discharge of patients to the community where they some-x Foreword

times had poorer care than in the hospital. It often lead to rigidities in staffing patterns and an inability to engage in staff substitutions that allowed more innovative practice. It often put scarce funds in upgrading physical facilities while patients were left with little real treatment. It reinforced investment in mental hospitals just at the time when it was becoming apparent that it was essential that public resources follow patients into the community. And once lawyers left the involuntary settings of the hospital they were far less effective in developing legal theories that protected and enhanced the interests of voluntary clients in community mental health care.

Having said all this, it is still my view that mental health legal activism substantially improved mental health care. Patients were often undertreated in the community, but one could find few clients in Alabama or elsewhere who were not happier with life in the community or who preferred to return to the hospital. Mental health funding has remained a persistent problem but legal activism and judicial interventions probably have been major factors contributing to increased public mental health allocations. Moreover, no reasonable person can contest the idea of a decent minimal standard that no public system should be allowed to violate. Anyone with experience in America's public mental hospitals in these decades knows that there were just too many instances of neglect and inhumane and degrading care.

This volume tracing the trajectory of a class action lawsuit in a Texas Federal Court is a remarkable document of considerable value to those of us working to improve care for persons with mental illness. It is unusual in that it is open to the voices of a range of important participants: clients and their families, advocates, the court monitor, mental health commissioners affected by the lawsuit, mental health professionals in the Texas system, consultants and evaluators from outside the state, and the federal judge. The participants present varying perspectives on the lawsuit and have been affected differently by it. Many of the lessons to be learned come less from the individual presentations and more from pondering the complexities and uncertainties of mental illness, the conflicts and contradictions among the perceptions of actors, and the fact that there is almost nothing more difficult than understanding how to shape social change to achieve our intended purposes. It is evident that these are dedicated individuals with good intentions but they perceive and experience the world differently, in large part because of their different roles and responsibilities. By better understanding the basis of their varied experiences and viewpoints, we appreciate better how we might approach the next stage in a continuing pursuit.

Providing excellent services for persons with serious and persistent mental illness is an uphill battle. The clients are often the most disadvantaged people in our society suffering from the largest vulnerabilities and stigmatizing images. They and their advocates have difficulty competing with highly organized disease interest groups that have more resources, greater public sympathy, and the ability to present a more united front. There is much to be said for judicial oversight in these easily exploitable circumstances. There is need, however, to continue to seek the way that involved groups can work together more harmoniously and productively in the promotion of a shared agenda.

Acknowledgments

I specifically want to thank the Honorable Barefoot Sanders, Senior Judge of the Northern District of Texas. Without his commitment to the idea that government has responsibility for those who cannot adequately care for or advocate for themselves, R.A.J. v. TXMHMR Commissioner, the case that is the subject of this book, would not have been resolved successfully.

I want to thank each of the contributors to this book: David Axelrad, M.D., David Bell, Ph.D., Hazel Byers, Marilyn Clark, Patsy Cheyney, Mary Dees, Art Farley, M.D., Don A. Gilbert, M.B.A., Howard H. Goldman, M.D., Ph.D., E. R. Hayes, M.D., F.A.C.P., Genevieve Hearon, Douglas Heinrichs, M.D., Lyn Henderson, Felicia Korman, M.S.W., Marty Lumpkin, Ph.D., Charles McDonald, Ph.D., David Mechanic, Ph.D., Susan Medlin, Gary E. Miller, M.D., Cynthia Patton Duran, Bill Smith, Ph.D., and Anne Mathews Younes, Ed.D. They have contributed their own perspectives about the implementation of this lawsuit. It is through the eyes of these participants that the reader can gain a greater sense of the complexity, adversarial nature, and ultimate humanity of the issues of this case.

I also want to acknowledge the participation of Martha Boston, James Peden, M.D., John Bateman, M.D., Deborah Peel, M.D., Nina Muse, M.D., George Gray, Nadine Jay, Raymond Leidig, M.D., Stephen Shanfield, M.D., and Andrew Barrick of the Civil Rights Division of the United States Department of Justice, which served as amicus curae.

The following attorneys diligently represented the Plaintiffs: Roger Getty, Laura Smith, Margo Michaels, Randall Chapman, John Heike, and Edward Cloutman, III.

The Texas Attorney General's Office was ably represented by Martha Allen, Jerry Covington, Phillip Durst, Patrick Weisman, Toni Hunter, Dennis Garza, Suzanne Marshall, Donna Hamilton, and Sarah Anderson.

I want to thank Dwight Spears and Donna Cox for years of service and commitment to the lawsuit and Wendy Wright for voluntarily editing the manuscript. Finally, I want to thank my wife, Mary, who survived the R.A.J. lawsuit with me for fifteen years with humor, consternation, anger, pride, hope, and a sense of awe that anything so worthwhile could be so hard to do.

State Hospital Reform

Chapter 1

Reminiscences

David Bell, Patsy Cheyney, Mary Dees,
Susan Medlin, and Anonymous

In 1974 a class action lawsuit was filed in a Texas Federal Court aimed at improving the living conditions in the state's eight psychiatric hospitals. Filed at a time of liberal interpretations of the legal rights of individuals, the goals of the litigation were to reform institutions in such a way that people would be protected, receive adequate psychiatric treatment, and upon discharge would be cared for adequately in the community. During the years when the State of Texas attempted to comply with the requirements of the suit, the political climate changed. Legal decisions moved from liberal interpretations of patients' rights to more conservative interpretations which questioned whether states needed to provide such care and treatment. However, efforts to comply with the original requirements of the court case went on and in 1997 this case was dismissed from the jurisdiction of the federal court as having achieved many of its original goals.

The purpose of this book is to tell the story of a major class action lawsuit in Texas aimed at improving the living conditions of patients in the state's eight psychiatric hospitals. At issue was the belief that the constitutional right of these patients were being violated and that they were subjected to inadequate treatment and put at risk of physical harm. The purpose of the lawsuit was to improve conditions in the hospital and in essence to reform a large state bureaucracy. The story contains drama, intrigue, politics, bureaucratic responses of government, and the despair of patients who are disenfranchised, misunderstood, and who, until recently, had nobody to advocate for them.

The following vignettes represent the memories of people who had experiences with the Texas state hospitals from 1974 to the present time. These experiences illustrate changes in conditions over the years.

4   State Hospital Reform: Why Was It So Hard to Accomplish?

Terrell State Hospital, 1974 David Bell, Ph.D.

I went to work at Terrell State Hospital on December 15, 1975. I had just completed a partial internship at a training hospital in Indiana and needed thirty more days to complete the required number of hours. No other facility was interested in a doctoral intern for thirty days, but Terrell was, as the R.A.J. lawsuit had just been filed and there was some interest in beginning to deal with the issues. Little did I know that I would be involved in a variety of ways with this lawsuit for the next twenty years.

After thirty days spent doing psychological evaluations, I was offered a job helping start up a program for mentally retarded persons. The first part of the job was to assess the number of mentally retarded persons and to get some estimate of their problems. This took me to almost every ward at Terrell, where I saw first hand the conditions there.

The patient areas were large, open "bays" with as many as twenty beds per bay and as little as one foot between the individual beds. The bays were separated by low walls which afforded no privacy. Each patient had a "night stand" with a 2" X 6" X 10" drawer which was used for personal articles. Beds were also in the halls and some areas which were meant as conference rooms also contained beds. The hospital was badly overcrowded, and patients were not separated by diagnosis, problems, or level of functioning. Patients wandered about the wards and grounds. The smell was of urine, cigar smoke, and dirty hair. Patients were given cigars as the lower sales tax made them cheaper than cigarettes. Smoking was universal in the wards. In the evenings, patients lined up naked to be bathed, showered, or actually hosed off in the showers. Some patients were restrained in beds, chairs, or to support columns in the wards. Mentally retarded persons of all levels were found in every ward. Following are examples of the type of patients I found:

> Sally who had no use of her lower limbs but had tremendous upper body strength which she used to drag herself around, on and off buses, and generally wherever she wanted to go. She had no language except grunts, groans, and growls. She was very aggressive, probably for self protection. She bit herself, and hit, kicked, and bit others. She slept on a mattress on the floor because it was easier to get on and off of. The staff was afraid of her and did not believe

that there was anything that could be done for her. She was in no training or activities, but she received large doses of antipsychotics, to control her behavior, which were ineffective as she was not psychotic.

Bobby, an adult autistic, walked around with every muscle tensed. He engaged in ritualistic behaviors such as hitting his hand and chest, which were red and raw. He frequently uttered in a bizarre voice, "Want some more hamburgers, want some more chocolate cake." He was often naked and masturbating, and had been restrained to a post. When clothed, Bobby wore white, tough coveralls backwards so they could not be easily removed. Because Bobby was very aggressive and dangerous, the staff was afraid of him. He was in no activities and received very large doses of two or three antipsychotics which were ineffective.

Sarah, a moderately retarded woman who was severely self abusive, was in restraints twenty-four hours per day. Sarah had split her skin open so many times that the tissue on her forehead was "granulated" and attempts at stitches pulled through as if through paper. When I met her, she was on the medical and surgical unit, having deliberately broken her arm. She was in a cast that covered her torso from neck to waist, with her arm held by a rod away from her body. She had already broken the cast and rebroke the arm once. Sarah was in no activities or training programs and was on large doses of antipsychotics, though she was not psychotic and the drugs were ineffective.

R.A.J. was on a ward where he was permanently housed in a seclusion room with a bed, a nightstand, and a table and chairs. He was aggressive and dangerous. Attempts made to bring him out were met with viscous attacks. Placing him in seclusion had begun as a temporary solution but then had become a permanent situation. The staff, especially one psychologist, was very concerned about R.A.J. I was requested to develop a program to get him out of the seclusion room, which did not occur because he was moved away from Terrell, being the main plaintiff in the suit.

Susan was totally blind and naked. She was kept in a seclusion room to prevent her attacks on others. She was on no training programs and took antipsychotics which had no effect. After moving to the new "Center for Human Development," a program for mentally retarded persons, she was kept out of seclusion and rather quickly learned her way about the ward.

Jesse was in a seclusion room on the medical and surgical unit, having ruined her throat by swallowing a caustic cleaning chemical. Her drinking had to be controlled because of the throat damage and the only way to do this, according to the staff, was to keep her in an empty room permanently. She was in no programs or training to alter any behaviors. She died in seclusion.

Ben, although deaf, was very strong and physically healthy and only mildly retarded. He sought the company of others and was friendly but very demanding when he was not understood. He was unable to communicate by signing because no one on the staff knew how to sign.

Marjorie had been hospitalized very young and was now in her late 40's. Her family was from Czechoslovakia and when she was committed, she did not speak English. No one on the staff when she was a child spoke Czech, and she had remained hospitalized as Mentally Retarded. She, like most of the mentally retarded at the hospitals, had developed many aggressive behaviors as a self protective strategy.

Daisy stood in the middle of the day room crying at an ear splitting level until she was give a soft drink, and then stopped until she was thirsty again. She was on no programs or training, and was on a dose of antipsychotics.

Ralph was a dangerous, aggressive, and very strong mentally retarded teenager. He often attacked other patients and staff, once pushing an elderly patient who fell and later died. Ralph knocked me unconscious once by butting me in the cheek. I strongly suspected that Ralph was badly abused by the night staff in revenge for his aggressive behavior.

There are numerous others. Over 200 were classified as Mentally Retarded based on a low IQ on a test called the Quick Test, which requires five minutes to administer. We began behavior therapy programs which generally worked very well and resulted in vast improvements. Most are now discharged to private placements or state schools.

When a patient came into the hospital, the ward physician wrote "routine" orders on a card. A very large percentage of these cards were identical. They contained orders for Thorazine, Stelazine, (both routine and p.r.n. for aggression) and p.r.n. seclusion, as well as aspirin, Milk of Magnesia, and other medicines which might be needed. If the Thorazine and Stelazine did not control behavior, additional orders would be written for Prolixin or Haldol. Many patients were on multiple antipsychotics in large doses, and it was unusual for medications to be reduced. When the Mentally Retarded were brought into one program, about two thirds of them were on antiseizure medications as a "preventative." Records were so sketchy that it was impossible to determine a seizure history. As our doctor, a retired OB/GYN, began reducing and discontinuing these, most patients did not have seizures, meaning they had probably never had a seizure disorder in the first place. Side effects included addiction to Phenobarbital and severe gum overgrowth from Dilantin. Many patients had mild to severe tardive dyskinesia, which was due to long years on high doses of antipsychotics, for which there was no treatment. There was a nearly universal belief among the physicians that multiple antipsychotics were completely necessary for these patients. When rulings began to be made about polypharmacy, most physicians were outraged, claiming that there would be chaos and regression by nearly all patients. This idea was not confirmed; many patients functioned better on lower doses of single medications, and many "psychotic" patients were not psychotic. The medicines were functioning as somewhat ineffective behavioral control devices.

Dr. S's prescription for out of control behavior was "rapid tranquilization: give 10 mg. of Haldol every thirty minutes till he is ataxic, then back off 10 mg. for the daily dose." Behavior problems were handled via what Dr. M. called: "The old 1-2-3: Thorazine, Stelazine, and Lock 'em up." There were no behavioral therapy programs, though there had been in the past. Self abusive and aggressive behaviors were rampant; mentally retarded persons were victimized by other patients and most would fight if approached. Using simple time out and personal restraint programs for brief periods quickly reduced aggression to manageable levels, but there was no program for control of aggressive behavior. One newly transferred aide walked about with a rolled up towel around his neck. Dr. M. saw this and became very angry, telling the man to get rid of the towel. I did not understand and when I quizzed Dr. M. he told me that the towel was to be used to "choke down" unruly patients.

Activities were conducted by the Central Rehabilitation staff, consisting of cheerful and enthusiastic persons who did recreational activities and occupational therapy, mainly crafts such as painting, weaving, and music. The rationale for the groups seemed to be that it afforded an opportunity to get the patients off the ward and doing something that hopefully they enjoyed and were willing to do. Higher functioning patients were given work assignments. Bus rides into town were popular: Jessie's twin sister Jane, who had been in a hospital in China, had one useful phrase, "Big bus ride to Shag Hi?"

There were numerous patients who were basically boarded. They had outside privileges and stayed off the wards most of the day, frequenting the canteen, the benches around the grounds, and sometimes the retired dairy barn, a popular romantic trysting place which was, sadly, torn down. Some traded sexual favors for cigarettes or 6 packs of soft drinks. Caffeinism was common. Many seizure patients drank tremendous amounts of coffee and soft drinks containing caffeine, though it became known that caffeine lowered the seizure threshold.

The weekly cardex meeting was the sole treatment review. The ward physician flipped through the green cards and chanted a litany: "No Change, No Change, No Change..."

After the suit was filed, there were serious efforts to begin training and rehabilitation, to have meaningful treatment reviews, to write new individualized treatment plans, and to reduce and/or change medications. However, the hospital still was understaffed and overcrowded so there were limits on what could be done. The attitude of the hospital and most staff towards the R.A.J. lawsuit was one of fear, hostility, and paranoia. Some of the staff, however, recognized that the lawsuit would bring pressure on the state legislature to provide necessary funds to provide at least basic treatment. Many resources were diverted to deal with the problem of mentally retarded persons in the hospital, and the process of change had begun.

Reminiscences   9

San Antonio State Hospital, 1978–1992, Patsy Cheyney

My youngest son celebrated his eighteenth birthday in the Bexar County Hospital. It was 1978, and he had broken a foot jumping from a second-story window, running from a deputy trying to take him to the San Antonio State Hospital for his second commitment. His diagnosis was paranoid schizophrenia.

By the early 1980's he was severely ill, his prognosis in the bottom quarter for recovery. He was missing for about a year; then the state hospital discharged or furloughed him as fast as he was committed. He became increasingly dangerous not only to himself, but to the community which seemed quite unable to cope with him. One morning in 1983, I decided that somebody, somewhere, was going to have to take some responsibility and it looked like that somebody was going to be me.

While he was missing, Andrew had walked a lot and had developed blisters on his feet. We were told later that when he was picked up he had decided that he had devils in his body and had tried to drive them out by cauterizing the blisters with a cigarette lighter. Several persons had refused even minimal assistance, and I swore that nobody was ever going to treat my child like that again.

Two other grown children shared my rented apartment and we took a vote. Unanimously, we voted that we were going to do whatever it took to get protection for, and from, Andrew. I had had previous organizing experience and we began to look for help. At a FAIR family support group we met other families who already knew of the existence of the NAMI movement and wanted to organize a local affiliate, but did not know how. I did the charter and the I.R.S. exemption, and by 1984 we were up and running. Of the first ten charter members, one was a stabilized manic-depressive and the other nine were relatives of schizophrenic patients in the state hospital.

We had already learned of the existence of two major legislative committees meeting regularly in Austin, one to draft a mental health code and the other to reorganize the mental health system. We began attending and met Dave Pharis and other state leaders.

On the oversight committee we encountered the attitude that schizophrenics were of no economic value to the state and should be put on the street in the full knowledge that they would die of exposure, starvation, or mistreatment. We were extremely angry, made no less so by an attitude which candidly favored allowing our family members to die as an economic inconvenience to the state. My daughter, Rachel, recalls those years succinctly. "The R.A.J. lawsuit was what gave us hope," she said. "Dave Pharis made us feel like there was somebody on our side."

In 1984, our concern was not over details of treatment—indeed, we did not know enough about modern medical treatment to worry about it. We looked only to creating a system that would guarantee enough sanctuary to keep our children alive until tomorrow. We knew well enough that schizophrenia was incurable. We fought for the "deterioration clause" and bitterly opposed the "single portal of entry" concept. We were outspoken.

By late 1984 TEXAMI was chartered. Genevieve Hearon of Austin had brought the concept to the state and had done most of the original organizing. I helped with the charter and I.R.S. exemption; Rachel put out the very first typewritten newsletter; Houston's AMI organized the first state convention. Trying to remember how we interacted with R.A.J. during those years, I asked a member from another AMI to refresh my memory. "You ought to remember!" she said. "Rachel had something about R.A.J. in practically every single newsletter!"

SAAMI got its first major publicity with its Christmas memorial service for the homeless mentally ill. We averaged about twenty-five deaths in 1984 and several years thereafter, and the score would have been worse had San Antonio not been blessed with a sub-tropical climate. We measured our gains by the drop in our death rate.

"We're like a group under siege," I testified during those years. "In wartime, the first thing you worry about is keeping your population alive until tomorrow. The day after tomorrow you worry about your committees."

Also in 1984 two major television stations did series on deinstitutionalization. Our family and two others were featured. Asked by a reporter to count the number of times Andrew had been committed, I said I had lost track somewhere between fifteen and twenty.

During the same time frame I sent an official "Notice to Sue" on attorney's letterhead, certified mail, to the superintendent at SASH, threatening to sue if Andrew were again released unstablized. That pretty much solved the commitment problem. He remained in the hospital system for about the next ten years, ultimately doing three terms in the maximum security unit at Rusk under writs of "manifest dangerousness" and another year on PICU, drugged almost to unconsciousness. "I like Rusk," said Andrew. "They have enough staff to keep the bad angels away." In terms of medical treatment, it was probably abominable; the hospital did, however, manage to keep him alive until Clozapine. Some of our families did not accomplish that degree of success.

Locally and statewide we wrote letters, made speeches, published newsletters, collared legislators, established coalitions — and filed complaints with R.A.J. In 1985 TEXAMI monitored requests for crisis care and developed an inventory of services; in 1986, we submitted a survey of needs to a legislative review commission with a list of twenty-five issues including discharge planning, still a major issue in this county. As R.A.J. findings were published and court orders issued, we used them to back up our testimony before legislative committees.

Locally, the city government had applied for H.U.D. grants for the homeless and, when those large shelters opened, our death rate declined. For the first time, we began to involve ourselves directly in service provision, and subsequently opened a twenty unit housing project for the long-term mentally ill. In 1994 a twenty-four unit project was under contract, and other AMIs had also received grants.

By 1989 it was obvious that court intervention could do little to improve continuity of care and discharge planning, but the publicity afforded comments of the court monitor continued to help build public opinion. As more and more Republicans were appointed to the appellate courts and concepts of federalism and states' rights began to reassert themselves, it became increasingly obvious that further successes would have to be based on negotiation. The only incentive for TXMHMR to negotiate was the need for legislative funding.

When plans to have consultants for the R.A.J. monitoring team were announced, I was very interested. Disappointed though I was with the failure of the federal government to enforce its orders, I nevertheless felt that all possible use should be made of the R.A.J. vehicle while it was available. When I was asked to participate I jumped at the chance. Its maximum impact was clearly in the area of peer review, where the insistence of physicians on improving diagnoses and treatments had a clearly discernible effect.

Such abstract legal concepts as procedural due process, culpable intents, distinctions between courts of inquiry and courts at law, "corpus delicti," and differences in standards of proof between criminal and tort cases were generally foreign to most of the consultants and had not been well-thought-out in advance; thus, the teams generally were not as well equipped to deal with them as they were medical issues. Concepts of natural rights and natural law were rampant—"The hospital should have done thus-and-so because it was the right thing to do!" "I just don't think that's right!" "They have a right to do that!" Hospitals adamantly opposed any attempt to modify their usual procedures, which were, in my opinion, about 400 years out-of-date.

As an attorney, I viewed such abstract issues as being especially amenable to redress in the court system and was quite disappointed in the results, but by 1993 it was too late to remedy this problem. The reluctance of the Bar in general to address the issues certainly contributed to the difficulties encountered.

During 1991 Andrew was tried on Clozapine, and about two years later was discharged to the Fairwether Lodge program, where he happily remains to this day, as pleasant, civil, hard-working, reliable, and friendly as if he had never heard of Rusk.

In 1993, expressing frustration to a psychiatrist traveling with me, I commented that professionals can address a narrow problem and go home and forget about it; family members have to develop a complete new system of social institutions—in effect, build a new life. "Don't worry about it; there's nothing you can do," he advised me kindly. I snorted, slammed the car door, went home, and began drafting what subsequently became subdivision "k" of the "abuse and neglect" bill in the 72nd legislature. Two years later, no longer consulting but still advocating, I drafted HB 1495, providing for improved notice of commitment hearings.

In the meantime, Rachel had taken her master's in social work; my oldest son had gone to medical school; and every member of the family, including my former husband and his second wife, in-laws, grandparents, aunts, uncles, cousins, and "significant others," stood behind our original decision. "Anybody that says 'dysfunctional family' never met us," we joked. "We can function just fine!" And we do.

Austin State Hospital, 1982, Mary Dees

Being unaware of the extent of the conditions that prompted that R.A.J. lawsuit in 1974, I will not be able to compare my later experience of 1982 as being the same or worse. I will, however, describe the condition of one of the state hospitals in 1982, and conditions at that same hospital that I recorded through my involvement with the Quality Service Oversight Statewide Team in 1994.

My initial experience with the TXMHMR system started when my private health insurance ran out in the early part of 1982. Following a drug overdose, I was very reluctantly, and civilly, entrusted to the care of one of the eight state mental hospitals in Texas. At the time of my admission and consequent six month stay, I have no memory of being informed of my rights or of the process to report rights violations or abuse and neglect allegations. Nor did I know that I was a plaintiff in a civil lawsuit, or that the hospital was a defendant. For the first three days of my stay, I was in a unit designated for residents from Houston, and although it was not at all like the inside of a private hospital, it was a familiar hospital-type setting. On day three, they (whoever "they" were) decided that they had made a mistake, and I was transferred to what was referred to as Capital A & B Unit. I was convinced I had been taken to either the prison section or Hell, but under no circumstance could I be in a hospital anymore.

The appearance of the day room was the first tell-tale sign that something was drastically wrong. The walls were concrete block painted with bright red and orange, with matching orange plastic barrel-type chairs lined up in rows facing a caged television secured high above eye-level on the wall. The nurses' station was enclosed with glass and bars. I wasn't sure if that was for the protection of the nurses or patients, as both looked equally dangerous. Staff were yelling at patients and the latter were either wandering aimlessly about the room or were yelling, screaming, or fighting, which resulted in four or five staff knocking them to the floor and dragging them to what I would later call their little private room, where they would stay sometimes for three and more days. During that time, they could be heard yelling, crying, screaming, or banging the wooden and/or glass window in the door.

My orientation to the Unit consisted of being warned by both staff and patients not to go to the laundry room, a.k.a. "The Sex Room."

The dorm, or sleeping area, consisted of rows of beds with bare mattresses, having no walls, and therefore, no privacy. The bathing room consisted of a large area with shower stalls, and a couple of tubs with no curtains.

Day number four validated my worst fear: I was in prison. The judge had sentenced me for thirty days, which was later extended to ninety. None of the staff explained to me that I could be released pending improvement. At one point, the attorney even discouraged me from attending the court proceedings. I would lose despite the fact that I was doing really well and was starting to act like a human being.

For four out of six months, my treatment consisted of being tied down in a four-point restraining bed in the day room. This left me helpless to ward off the male patients, who would touch and stroke me. I was also witness to cockroach races and male patients urinating on the floor nearby. The staff were no more hospitable: on one occasion I was subjected to a large heavy staff member sitting on me; on another occasion, I was tied to a chair secured to a cement support column in the middle of the day-room, with the staff threatening to photograph me for the purpose of showing my family and friends how stupid I looked. I never reported any of these altercations because I viewed myself as a prisoner and expected bad treatment. One event from this painful part of my life exemplifies the attitude of the staff, and the credibility the patients had at the hospitals at the time. One night I was awakened by a man standing over my bed and the smell of something burning. Someone had set fire to the mattress next to mine. I ran to the nurses' station to tell them what was happening, and was told to go back to bed and to stop making up stories.

I could continue, but I think I have painted a gloomy enough picture. I am happy to say that the R.A.J. lawsuit has dramatically changed the physical aspects of the hospital. Today, that same state hospital could compete with most local private mental hospitals. Patients, upon admission, are now told of their rights. Both the R.A.J. Settlement as well as patient rights are posted in high traffic areas of the hospital in large, very readable print. Sleeping and bathing areas are now providing some level of privacy. Patients are no longer being tied to their beds in the day room and they are usually not drugged to the point that they resemble the cast from a horror movie. The noise levels have decreased, maybe not enough to satisfy me, but a significant amount. Patients are now encouraged to hang up pictures and are able to have personal belongings in their rooms. Take-downs and seclusions, in my opinion, have been drastically reduced. I am not sure if this is due to R.A.J. or new drugs, or both. The television is no longer caged on the wall, and in some areas there are stereos and aquariums.

More important is what I consider to be a shift in staff attitude. I sense that rather than disdain and dread, an attitude of pride and compassion is starting to emerge. Staff are talking to, and I believe more often than not, listening to patients.

It is not hard to see that I started my role as a consultant out of rage, anger, and more importantly a deep hurt that needed to be resolved. In my willingness to both change the system and stop my internal sense of emotional pain, I took chances, asked questions, and took the time to listen to what was being said. I spent hours reading rules, asking questions, and searching ways to fix the problems, and I did so as a very angry and hurt consumer. As I learned more, and listened more, I began to see differently with a broader vision for what was the answer for consumers, not just me. On at least two separate occasions I had limitations set upon my input which in my opinion protected me from harm in a very consumer empowerment sensitive way. It is very important for me to hear that the R.A.J. lawsuit has come to and end, not that it means that the system does not have problems. However, it marks an end to the anger driven consumer I started out as and the beginning of a consultant who looks at people issues.

Austin State Hospital, 1994, Susan Medlin

The following is a summary account of my experience and observations as a patient at Austin State Hospital in 1994. First, I wish to commend the direct care staff who were respectful and polite in their interactions with me during my treatment. I also received good clinical care. The doctor was responsive to my needs and accommodating in working with my private psychiatrist while I was experiencing a medication related crisis. However, I did observe a number of conditions which compromised the dignity and respect of patients on the ward. Most of the problems I observed arose from one or more of the following sets of circumstances: dysfunctional policies set by the administration, overcrowding, and shortage of staff to cope with the problems resulting from the overcrowded environment.

16   State Hospital Reform: Why Was It So Hard to Accomplish?

Perhaps the most comprehensive source of problems was the combination of overcrowding and an administrative policy that did not adequately provide enough staff members per shift to work with the number of patients on the ward. One result which was demeaning to women patients was that the shower attendants had to leave the doors open to the showers in case they had to be called out or needed to summon another staff member in an emergency. The doors remained open despite the fact that there were male staff on the ward. Another problem was that despite the private bedrooms for patients who are likely to disturb others at night, the ward's crowded condition resulted in there being at least one patient in each bedroom who would continuously disturb others throughout the night. Each communal bedroom holds five patients. One of the patients in my bedroom had a habit of waking up at 4:00 a.m. on the dot loudly singing hymns. The staff responded by administering medication which unfortunately was not effective until our entire room was soundly awake.

There were other difficulties associated with overcrowding and under staffing. Because there were not enough staff for any one member to be solely assigned to one-on-one duty, the person under observation was sometimes compelled to follow the staff member around as he conducted his regular duties as necessary. This also kept the one-on-one patient from being able to attend classes, which is in conflict with hospital policy. Furthermore, since the staff frequently swapped out for one-on-one duty, most of the patients on the ward shared the inconvenience of waiting long periods to access their personal belongings which were locked up in closets in their locked bedrooms. Actually, this was also true when there were no patients on one-on-one precautions: There was simply not enough staff.

Additional problems related to administrative policy were apparent in the use of time out as a restrictive intervention and in the requirement that patients remain in the day room virtually at all times. Exceptions to remaining in the day room were minimal, including a brief rest period after lunch and a few short breaks. The main activity was attending classes. However, there were no classes on Friday and patients were left with few productive options. This lack of activity or outlet not only erodes respect but is also counterproductive to treatment. Although time out is intended as a voluntary decision by an individual to take some time alone to calm down, it was inappropriately utilized as an involuntary intervention in which a person's egress from a room is prevented. This is the official hospital policy, although TXMHMR's Consumer Services and Rights Protection has interpreted this as seclusion. Staff were not appropriately trained in the use of physical restraint procedures. I also witnessed a woman being dragged down the hall to the seclusion room.

These problems are not only detrimental to the respect and dignity of individuals in psychiatric hospital care, but also to the quality of care that they receive while in the hospital. The system would be more effective fiscally and therapeutically if patients received optimal care and were able to leave earlier as a result.

Austin State Hospital, 1994, Anonymous

On a winter day in 1994, I phoned both my psychiatrist and my counselor in hopes of being able to meet with one or the other that day because I was feeling rather desperate and was trying to do something positive to help myself. Messages were left on both answering machines requesting a call back as soon as possible. Eventually the psychiatrist's receptionist called me back and said she would page my doctor and have him call me. Quite some time passed with no calls, so I rang her again. I was becoming increasingly panicked at having received no response. The receptionist told me she would again page my doctor, but advised that I should go to a local private psychiatric hospital. I said I didn't feel that I needed such an extreme solution and would at least like to have an opportunity to discuss it with my doctor first, especially because during our last visit two days prior we had agreed that a hospital was not the place for me. An hour and a half went by without a call, so my boyfriend and I decided that a walk would do us some good.

Upon returning to my apartment thirty to forty-five minutes later, I was greeted by four policemen dressed in full riot gear, complete with helmets, goggles, and billy clubs, and three or four EMS men. It appeared as though they were going to bust my door down. My instinct was to not deal with these people, but my boyfriend said he would take care of things to disperse them and tell them that there was no problem. They had been waiting there fifteen minutes. They wouldn't go away. Apparently the receptionist had phoned the EMS when I wasn't there to receive her call. The EMS looked at and re-bandaged a cut I had made on my wrist three or four days earlier (my doctor was aware of this cut), I signed a waiver saying I refused medical attention and did not want to go with them. The EMS began to leave.

A policeman was using my phone. My body was trembling at the chaos. My boyfriend said he would see the police out. I went into the bathroom and shut the door to wait. This action brought on pounding on the door, handcuffs, a ride in the back of a police car, and a drive to a mysterious destination for a reason unrevealed. They had taken me to the State Hospital.

I went through the preliminaries and was cooperative and honest with the admissions doctor. "Essentially," I said, "it was a case of miscommunication and poor timing". I made repeated requests that he phone my psychiatrist so that he could be consulted. This request was ignored and diverted repeatedly. Ultimately, I was involuntarily committed for at least a twenty-four hour "critical care crisis watch." Though I inquired, I was not told what this meant. I inquired as to my rights and all I was told was that I have no choice in the matter. After twenty-four hours, I could appeal the commitment in front of a judge—a process which could take weeks. I again stated my objection to being hospitalized and requested that my doctor be contacted. He was contacted at last. By this point I was very upset. Apparently my doctor concurred with the admissions doctor that I should be committed, although I have no way of knowing whether or not this is true. I was given my toothbrush bag and taken to the ward.

Many of my belongings were taken from me, including my medicine, shoelaces and lighter, "as a protective measure." I was searched in front of other ward members. I was instructed to shower, but was not allowed privacy from the male staff. Supposedly this is normal, but it made me terribly uncomfortable and I felt like a criminal. I was not allowed to move from one chair to another or go to my bed without an O.K. from staff. I was accompanied to the toilet and watched, making it very difficult to do my business, and was humiliated and cursed at by a female staff because of this difficulty. I was not given a copy of my rights, any information on the lawsuit, or any idea what was expected of me until I was released from the hospital. I received no counseling or advice. I was not allowed to participate in classes other ward mates attended. After getting into bed, I was threatened with a strip search because "somebody had been smoking in a bathroom down the hall." As I wasn't allowed anywhere on my own, I didn't see how it could possibly be me. This escaped the reasoning of the staff. I was spared the strip search, but was prevented from sleeping by having a flashlight shined in my eyes every fifteen minutes by a female staff. I was not protected from other female patients, many of whom were violent, threatening and harassing. I had items of little value to none but myself stolen from me by patients. There was no safe place provided to put these things. I was not allowed to exercise. When allowed outside, I was confined to a three-foot by six-foot area in front of the door. The men were allowed out at the same time as the women. I was not protected from these men, two of whom were threatening and one of whom insisted on touching my body and rubbing his body against mine. The male staff would do nothing to intercede. I was insulted, ridiculed and humiliated repeatedly, mainly by the female staff, but also by a physician who performed a physical exam. He made an offensive comment during a breast exam. My special dietary needs were ignored. I was not allowed to take my medicine as my doctor has prescribed, and was therefore over-medicated in terms of sedation and under-medicated in terms of anti-depressants. We were all treated as bad-seed, learning-disabled, barely-human children who were incapable of the most basic brain functions and motor skills, and who responded only to condescension, insults, and threats. I saw an actual psychiatric doctor for one less-than-five-minute interview, immediately prior to my discharge. As far as I could tell, the purpose of this interview was merely to dissolve the state of any legal responsibility for my safety or well-being in order to make room for incoming patients. I saw my "social worker" for three minutes—to sign my release paperwork. My stay was approximately twenty-seven hours. I came out more depressed, anxious, paranoid, and suicidal than I went in.

The upshot is that I feel that the hospital is using its very limited resources in a very unproductive manner. The staff have no training in counseling, psychology, or abuse victims whatsoever. Few, if any, have been to college, and many have not completed high-school. They are minimum-wage, unskilled laborers, who receive less formal orientation into the job than nighttime doormen at apartment complexes. During my stay, there were at least four night staff, and six to seven day staff. They apparently had little to do, as they sat around playing cards, eating burgers, and making fun of the patients. They were all getting paid to do this at the expense of not being able to have even one trained counselor on hand. Why not get rid of two staff and hire someone who can be supportive and helpful, or at least aware? Or why not offer comp time to the teachers of the purportedly helpful (I don't know, as I wasn't allowed to attend any) mental health classes if they spend additional time with the patients in the actual ward? This would not cost much, and would provide much needed integration, which is essential in learning and adopting new coping skills.

Finally, I feel that it would be much more manageable for the state, and better for the well-being of the patients, if some distinction were made between those patients that are violent, uncontrollable and psychotic, and those that are merely neurotic and depressed. Even a separation by rooms or schedules would have made my stay much less terrorizing. I understand that at one time there was a separate facility to house or care for these "intermediate crisis" patients. The lack of resources should not negate the necessity for this separation. Schedule and room assignment changes could considerably alleviate much of the tensions inherent in dealing with a disparate group of mental patients.

Vernon State Hospital, 1995, Anonymous

The employees we have come in contact with at Vernon State Hospital are not only efficient in their fields, but are also courteous and caring people, dedicated, and willing to readily help us in our needs. With our lives stressed from recent occurring events, their "caring" has truly been a "godsend" to us and needless to write we are appreciative, and are also appreciative of the care of our son. We realize now why Vernon State Hospital was apparently the first hospital to pass the monitoring regulations in regards to the R.A.J. lawsuit.

Our son was admitted to the psychiatric unit at Vernon State Hospital during August 1995, and after a medical crisis was transferred to a general hospital. We have been kept informed by phone calls on all issues affecting him. When we came to the general hospital to be with our son during the crisis of his illness a staff member met us there. Talking to her on the phone was always helpful to us and then meeting her, she reached out to offer more help. She even arranged for us to speak with the physician regarding our son's illness. The physician was kind enough to take time out of his busy schedule to speak with us.

The social worker has been most helpful, giving us information on phone numbers and just being there to assist us with answers to our questions, and always willing to take the time to do this.

The state hospital chaplain was very compassionate and kind, taking the time to come to the local hospital and offer encouragement and prayers; truly a spiritual uplift!

We were very much impressed by the security guards from the state hospital who alternated shifts at the general hospital. We expected these men to be very stern authoritarians but to our grateful surprise, they were caring individuals, doing their assigned jobs, but human enough to be understanding and kind.

Terrell in the 1990's, David Bell, Ph.D.

There have been numerous meaningful changes since the 1970's at Terrell and many other hospitals. Most of the mentally retarded persons who were there have moved on to other places, some much better. Persons with whom I have grappled on the floor for my own and other's protection now live in homes where they may live normal lives. They help with meals, do household chores, walk to the bus and go to work, in some cases. Others have moved to state schools. Sadly, in some cases, placements are not so therapeutic. I have seen many large "nursing homes" which house former Terrell patients. The environments, level of activities, and other features of these homes are not much better than those at Terrell in the 70's. Presumably, most are still not subjected to the misuses of medication and abuse that were relatively common, however, there is no good provision to insure adequate treatment with individualized treatment plans and the safeguards required at the hospitals.

When mentally retarded persons come to Terrell now, it is for treatment. Some remain, as they had so many psychiatric and behavior problems that no placements would take them.

The hospital has been extensively remodeled. There are now walls in patient bedrooms, affording some privacy. Clients have space for personal articles and the staff understands that patients have a right to personal property. Patients are in activities, though there is still a tendency to place them in large groups in recreation or other activities that may or may not be very helpful to the individuals being treated. There have been individual behavior modification programs, some quite dramatic, that have reduced and sometimes eliminated problem behaviors and lack of motivation. Individual behavior modification programs were used extensively in the 1980's but there is less use of these mechanisms today than previously. Staff members claim that the paperwork is too difficult and detailed to make such programs feasible.

The physical environment is much more modern and pleasant. All wards are no smoking, and patients are safer from attack by others. Patient abuse is greatly reduced by an aggressive advocacy system that investigates complaints. There is a an excellent clients' rights office with several staff members, including former patients who help insure patients' rights are observed. Restraint and seclusion are very much reduced, to a point where there have been a few problems with documentation; staff simply do not get enough "practice." In some cases, the routine use of seclusion for minor offenses, or for prolonged periods, is a fraction of what was in the past.

Patients now have an active treatment plan, which they are supposed to sign in agreement and which is periodically reviewed. Individual problems are addressed according to priority, and according to a "formulation," a statement by the treatment team of exactly how the patient got sick and what will be done to help him or her get better. "Routine" orders are minimal, and medications are individualized and only given via patient consent. There is a legal mechanism set up for medication refusal which allows each patient his or her day in court if he or she disagrees with the doctor. Polypharmacy, formerly rampant, is rare with antipsychotics and requires clinical review by another physician. Medical problems are attended to much more efficiently and in accordance with medical trends. Tardive dyskinesia is rare and taken very seriously, as it should be. Patient participation is the rule of the day, and quality oversight systems are in place with appropriate help and education for treatment team members who need it. Most significantly, patient population is down from over 2,000 to under 500.

There is still room for improvement. Behavior therapy needs to be used more in order to change behaviors which cause hospitalizations. The staff have become so tired of the paperwork involved that they simply do not wish to continue to do these programs. Rehabilitation therapies need to be more individualized, as there is still a tendency to force fit problems into standard groups. More rehabilitation therapists are needed to try to deal with this problem. There are few crisis beds available and those that are there prove that hospitalization can be prevented in many if not most cases. One program with which I am familiar, in a rural area, greatly reduces visits to Terrell by providing a few days of housing, medication management, and crisis stabilization. The quality of staff is greatly improved, but there is a need for improved compensation of professional staff and more education and relevant training for ward workers.

If quality oversight is shortchanged problems will return and there is some fear now the Department will reduce efforts at quality improvement. Once the pressure of the lawsuit is reduced the hospitals may be inclined to cut back or eliminate quality management systems, and the legislature may well reduce funding.

Chapter 2

May Our Tears Be Turned into Dancing

Genevieve Tarlton Hearon

My daughter's years in and out of state hospitals coincided with national mental health events and institutional reform lawsuits of the seventies and eighties. Her saga shows how one person's strength, loss and gradual improvement parallels large scale systems change. The Texas Department of Mental Health and Mental Retardation (TXMHMR) ran an inadequate hospital and community system in the mid-seventies and eighties. It not only crushed my daughter's spirit, but it almost physically killed her. Gemee experienced the great violations of patients rights that occurred in Texas hospitals, the gradual impact of the R.A.J. institutional reform lawsuit on her daily life, the improved hospital system and the growth of community services. Her story represents the ravages of thousands of individuals with schizophrenia who were committed to state hospitals.

Most family members and consumers of mental health services of the mid-seventies and eighties did not share their stories with policy makers. Many families were too ashamed of discrimination due to their loved one's mental illness and hid their faces with anonymity.

No one's energy should be wasted on being anonymous. Honest disclosure by family members and consumers captured policy makers' and legislators' attention in the mid-eighties and kept them from turning away. Personal stories of their constituents intensified the pressure of the R.A.J. lawsuit which the Legislatures of 1985, 1987, 1989 and 1991 desperately wanted "to get out of."

Fragmented hospital and community systems precipitated Gemee's greater incremental deterioration. Unplanned hospital discharges were abrupt. Gemee also experienced staff's encouragement of her independence as a push away from hospital treatment into predictable crisis on the streets and highways. She tried hard to survive without community supports that were not yet developed, and she was re-peatedly re-hospitalized or incarcerated in jails due to manifestations of her schizophrenia.

Her institutional years demonstrate that state hospital reforms did not happen steadily, silently or without considerable pain and tears. Stabilizing her symptoms of schizophrenia replaced her dream of becoming a professional ballerina which was the work of her youth. Her motivation to work plummeted with re-hospitalizations, her dream was lost forever and our learning to dream differently became a shared destination.

Concerned advocacy groups, champion legislators, national mental health events, the R.A.J. lawsuit and the media brought about public awareness. Legislatures gradually funded TXMHMR programs to ensure consumer rights to quality treatment, to improve professional standards and to implement programs with an emphasis on community support services.

We cannot lose the progress we have made. We cannot allow for the erosion of beneficial outcomes for consumers of mental health services. So, I tell my personal perspective of Gemee's story.

Gemee, born in 1957, was a full-term baby with a difficult breech delivery. We were in Waco, Texas where she grew into a healthy, imaginative, strong-minded and loving toddler. When Gemee was three, she described sunsets as "the sun is melting out." In that same year, 1960, Martin Burnbaum defined the Right to Treatment for individuals committed to state hospitals. We had moved to Washington, DC in 1959. Her sister, Tarlton, was born in 1961 and her brother Burney in September 1963. She enjoyed having a sister and brother. In January 1963 my husband, against my will, decided we were moving to Corpus Christi, Texas, my home town. By 1963, my interest in mental health had also formed and I recall that in that same year I proudly heard President Kennedy announce the National Mental Health Facilities Act.

Even though Gemee may have felt our stress when her brother Burney was diagnosed mentally retarded in 1964, and my husband and I divorced in 1966, she was accepting. When she was in the fourth grade in 1967, she made all "A"s to earn the privilege of taking ballet lessons. In 1968, she embraced my remarriage and the birth of her half-brother, Paul. Gemee was very successful through the 7th grade and completed her goals in dance, drama, piano, camping and science activities. Her ready smile lit up her classic face. She had a lovely graceful body and was never awkward.

In 1970, the first lawsuit on the right to treatment in state institutions, Wyatt v. Stickney, was filed in Alabama. In a talent show in Corpus Christi, 12-year-old Gemee danced on toe while a handsome young man played the theme to the movie "Love Story" on a baby grand piano. Women in the audience wept. This duet won the city-wide contest.

At age thirteen, Gemee often complained of splitting headaches. When the medical doctor ruled out organic causes, I took her to a psychologist who stated that we could return to a productive routine when we achieved "good mental health." I believed we could. I had a Master's Degree in Education, had studied various child and adolescent learning theories including Montessori, had opened three schools and a training center and was currently administering a very successful school for seventy children. I was more than familiar with the learning needs of children and adolescents. This therapist promoted the belief that positive parent-child relationships would resolve everything. I dealt with her adolescence and my reactions for years until the myth was shattered by understanding mental illness. Gemee began a cycle of running away from her splitting headaches.

After a scheduled summer visit with their father and step-mother in Miami in 1971, Gemee and Tarlton did not return to Corpus Christi as planned. I waited at the airport for my girls to get off the airplane, and they did not. I had no warning. Their father had begun a ten month legal struggle to change their custody to him and his wife. I went to Miami and fought. Gemee cried that Jesus talked out of her mouth saying she needed to stay with her father. I fought from my home in Corpus Christi and traveled back and forth to Miami, divorced Paul's father, hired, fired and hired Miami attorneys, but to no avail. A Florida judge granted custody to their father and his wife in June.

In 1972, Welch v. Likins, a right to treatment lawsuit, was filed in Minnesota. This case articulated the concept of the right to treatment in the least restrictive environment. In April, I placed Burney, age seven, into the care of the Corpus Christi State School for Mental Retardation.

I sold my school, let go seven staff and said good-bye to seventy children. Paul, age four, and I moved to Austin in December, to begin again. In January, 1973, I began working at the state capitol during the 140 day session as an administrative assistant for a state senator. After the session I worked for the joint House /Senate Committee on Prison Reform.

When Paul and I went to Miami for Easter 1974, Tarlton said Gemee was "different." Gemee's "poems" were incoherent clusters of imaginative words. That spring, her father moved from Miami to Atlanta with his wife, their son and Tarlton. Gemee called me from a Miami boarding school. She wanted to leave it and come home to dance. When she finished the school year, she'd won the Drama Award for her role as Anne Frank. I sent her a plane ticket for Austin.

She was fifteen when she returned. She completely distrusted me, saying we could never trust each other again because she had sided with her father during the custody battle. She was fearful and suffered splitting headaches. However, she still took private and group ballet lessons. She taught drama to elementary school pupils at a summer camp. Only her work ethic was intact. Once she was up to speed in her dancing, she was invited to become a member of the Austin Ballet Theater. Gemee was overjoyed.

In 1974 the Davis v. Watkins and the R.A.J. institutional reform lawsuits were filed respectively in Ohio and Texas. The R.A.J. lawsuit sought from TXMHMR guarantees for the protection of patients rights, their protection from harm, their right to consent to medication, their right to be treated with dignity and their right to adequate medical and psychiatric treatment.

In April 1974, Gemee ran away from a splitting headache after seeing the high school psychologist. In her abandoned room I sighed at the huge number of her well-worn pink toe shoes, accumulated since the mid-60's, which hung from her bedroom light fixture over her empty bed. Reams of her incoherent poetry and funky paintings filled a cedar chest. I remember Gemee's singing, from Janis Joplin's version of "Me and Bobby McGee," "Freedom's just another word for nothin' left to lose." I was haunted by Janis Joplin's early death.

In May I received a letter from Gemee. She was "hijacked" by a con-man to become a movie star. He bought her a bikini, drove her to Hollywood and left her. When she returned home, she was overweight, devastated and frightened. She sobbed over losing her ballet role in the Austin Ballet Theater due to her missing their practices. She wept often and uncontrollably. This went on for years.

Gemee accepted a psychologist who became our therapist. He believed that much of her emotional disturbance was caused by the trauma of her father's custody battle. That summer she ran away to Corpus Christi. Paul's father, her ex-step father, provided her with an apartment. She received a GED, went to Junior College for a semester and earned a few credits. She returned to me in Austin complaining about "mental problems." She refused to describe them and resumed her therapy with the psychologist. She worked as a file clerk for a state agency and also as a waitress. She hoped to go to college later. She, Paul and I really missed Tarlton.

From 1974 to 1976, her concentration would repeatedly deteriorate and she blamed her splitting headaches. Every two or three months we made a family visit to see Burney at the Corpus Christi State School. On one trip in 1975, she jumped out of the car as I drove and ran away. I didn't see her again until she was in the Austin State Hospital Adolescent Unit. She had been jailed, hospitalized in Houston and brought back to Austin. Later she told me she'd been with "a mountain man, Buck." Her therapist and I visited her at the hospital and he told me she'd have to change her peer relationships to make any headway in therapy. She was released to me after two days, and she began job hunting.

In 1975, the Dickson v. Sullivan lawsuit on the right to treatment for patients at St. Elizabeth's Hospital was filed in Washington, D.C. Gemee tried hard to be stable. I helped her get work as a page for the State Senate from January through May and as a cashier through the summer, a time when I was also looking for other employment. She was unreasonably controlling about what I wore for job interviews and critical of Paul's behavior. She suddenly ran away without an apparent cause. I later learned that her boyfriend took her to San Francisco. There, she became pregnant. He was arrested and sent to prison; she was abandoned and called me from Oregon. She arrived home with a young man who appeared to be as psychotic as she was. I had to leave them in our home while I took Paul to school and I went to work at the Texas Education Agency. Her therapist said she'd have to learn by the consequences of her actions and I'd have to be ready to pick up the pieces if I wanted to. Still I chased the mental health therapy myth. I had not yet learned that we were dealing with something more than the problems that parents can resolve.

In 1976, Brewster v. Dukasis was filed in Massachusetts. Plaintiffs claimed that they were being denied treatment in the least restrictive setting because community services were not available. The case focused on the development of such services. In another attempt to make sense out of her behavior, our good friend, Jerry, charted Gemee's biorhythms; I gave her extra support to offset her projected biorhythm clashes, she stabilized; then she ran away after Christmas. I began to think that something physical was the matter with her.

I later learned she had once again aligned herself with an older domineering male and gone to New York and Pennsylvania. When she returned to Austin in September, the police took her to the state hospital where she was committed for ninety days to Adult Services as she was now eighteen.

I passed through locked doors into an overcrowded smoke-filled room and saw a couple of aides watching the many male and female patients from a cage-like protected section; next to their cage, double swinging doors hid the dormitory, toilets and showers for women. An overpowering disinfectant smell and stale air permeated the building. The thirty-year-old heating and cooling system did not work. The poorly planned layout was dangerous; when females went to the bathroom they could be assaulted by males without the knowledge of staff. A large TV hung high on a wall blasting noise into the room, and nobody watched it. I saw several individuals try the water fountains that failed to work. A door opened to a hot and bare outdoor area that was fenced. A few patients wandered into the blazing sun to smoke and pace. Others aimlessly wandered about the noisy, smoke-filled, smelly ward. Some patients slumped in orange plastic chairs. The buzzer loudly announced the unlocking of the door. It did not make any difference who was entering, patients swarmed around any visitor to plead for some attention to meet their needs. They grabbed, touched and clung to me as I looked for Gemee, asking if I was their social worker or doctor.

Francisco rapidly spoke to me about his relationship with the King of Spain, an Asian artist with his pen and paper in hand slanted his body and slid across the floor, and a tiny African-American woman curled up in anyone's arms that would take her. Gemee came through the swinging doors of the dormitory complaining that she couldn't get anything for her constipation. She told me in elaborate detail and sincerity that one of her teeth transmitted the news about Patty Hearst, Charles Manson, and Jack and Bobby Kennedy. She also told staff. She later found pliers and pulled out that tooth. I took her off the hospital grounds to a private dentist. I found I had to take her to private doctors. She was not receiving adequate medical or dental treatment, yet hospital aides registered her to vote and took her to the polls where she voted for Jimmy Carter and the local sheriff.

Patients like Gemee were committed for a maximum of ninety days, although many were discharged or ran away after a shorter time. There was a high recidivism rate because the hospital doctors quickly discharged patients. Doctors gave them a short supply of medications. Without community supports mentally ill dischargees often forgot to take their medications, they ran out of them, stopped taking them or self-medicated with alcohol or street drugs. Deteriorating into psychosis, they drew the attention of the police who took them to jail or to the state hospital for another admission. At that time hospital staff did not refer a patient who was being discharged to any service outside the hospital. While the local mental health center served discharged patients, hospital staff did not refer patients to this center. As a result, patients deteriorated faster. They became psychotic sooner and returned to the hospital more quickly.

Because I live in Austin, I visited Gemee at the hospital daily and was familiar with the staff. On several occasions, I came for a visit to find Gemee had already been discharged to an older male I did not know. The hospital staff never asked her if she wanted me to know she was being discharged. I was angry and troubled. I wondered how many other families were experiencing this type of insensitivity.

Staff repeatedly set unrealistic goals for Gemee. They encouraged her to be independent of me, told her to get a job on her own, and they never counseled her about the self-destructive consequences of her habitually running away with exploitative men who raped her or unstable men who wanted to help her, but could not help themselves. At times, she took staff's encouragement of her independence to unrealistic extremes.

When her "independence" led to a return of her psychosis, she was readmitted by the same angry and overworked staff who had encouraged her "independence." They now humiliated her and she felt like a failure. Gemee constantly lost her personal belongings at the hospital. Staff routinely made excuses. Her clothes and other personal items were unaccountably "lost." Often Gemee bought them again from staff at the Hospital Thrift Store. My complaints were met with inertia and buck-passing. Staff morale was low, turnover was high and the pay was minimum. Staff constantly shifted blame for their actions to workers on other shifts, other patients, the laundry system, administrative rules, "Central Office" and the State Legislature for lack of funding for additional staff.

Another hospital reform lawsuit, Doe v. Kline, was filed in New Jersey in 1977.

In January 1977, Gemee found work as a Page for the State House of Representatives. Her new friend, a domineering hippie in his mid-thirties, paneled and carpeted a room and bath behind our carport for her. He gave her a second hand car. After the Legislative Session, she ran off to Puerto Rico with him. Years later she told me this was a drug run. When she returned, she had deteriorated and was re-hospitalized. After being discharged, she came home. Now the best job she could find was as a laundry sorter. Gemee's car was hit at an intersection. Fearful, she never drove again. Unexpectedly, she went to Baton Rouge, Louisiana where she worked as a waitress.

Baton Rouge law enforcement hospitalized her. A boy who was a friend to her brought her home in November. Gemee was very sick and needed to resume treatment if she was to stabilize. I took her to the Emergency Services at Brackenridge Hospital where she was examined, diagnosed for the first time as having schizophrenia and transferred by the police to the State Hospital. Bob, who would soon become my husband, and I followed her to Admissions. I wanted to be with her. We were brushed aside as the hospital staff whisked her away to the adult ward. As she was now 19, I was treated differently. Staff did not have to answer my questions about therapy, schedules and next steps. I was dismissed abruptly. Staff believed they were protecting the autonomy and confidentiality of the adult patient.

Tragically, the therapist Gemee had since 1974 died of brain cancer in September of 1977 while she was in Baton Rouge. I asked Dr. Jackson Day, the community's leading child and adolescent psychiatrist, to evaluate and treat her during this hospital stay and discharge. She accepted him, and he treated her for the next six years until he, too, died of brain cancer.

Because of adverse financial conditions, recruiting doctors for the state hospitals was difficult, and so staff doctors had to work double and triple shifts. Limited state-wide professional recruitment resulted in a heavy reliance on foreign doctors. I recognized the difficult conditions and their stress. Even so, the physicians' rudeness was appalling. They did not want to communicate with me, and I spoke their language fluently. Tarlton, Paul and I celebrated Gemee's 20th birthday in December 1977 with cake for all the patients on the ward who wanted a piece.

After her ninety days, Gemee was discharged and remained at home for several months. As I lay asleep the night before New Year's Eve, her current boyfriend tried to rape me. He was so drunk that I was able to push him away and find Gemee to warn her that he might go to her room. Very frightened, she voluntarily committed herself. Her private psychiatrist treated her with Prolixin; she continued seeing him after her next ninety days which was the first planned discharge she'd ever had. She made a friend, a woman named Rhonda who had physical disabilities. She took a job at Pizza Hut and lived in a nearby garage apartment. Prolixin had side effects; she could not see the smudges on the drinking glasses which was part of her job. She did not smell a dangerous gas leak at her apartment where I found her asleep. I called the gas company and moved her to Rhonda's trailer where she wanted to go and was welcome.

Her psychiatrist, Bob, I, and other family members patched together a support system which attempted to help Gemee to stay out of harm's way. Although tempted, she did not run away that year.

Legal efforts to settle the R.A.J. lawsuit continued to fail in 1977 and 1978.

In the winter of 1978, Gemee went to an Alcoholics Anonymous (AA) meeting. A thin, older, agitated man brought her home and announced he would save her; he did not believe in "drugs." She left with him immediately. Without medications she deteriorated into psychosis. After two weeks, he left her alone at a motel. The would-be rapist boyfriend called after I was home from work saying Gemee was sick and he would "drop her off." She came in more psychotic and pitiful than I'd ever seen. I took her directly to the state hospital. She had another birthday in the hospital and after ninety days was discharged, again without workable plans.

Congress passed and funded the National Plan for the Chronically Mentally Ill. Both President and Mrs. Carter had fought long and hard for its passage.

In 1979, she was re-hospitalized and disappeared again. Eventually, I found her living with a severely disabled cartoonist who also did not believe in medications. She was off of her medications, emaciated and very psychotic. Later she threw his furniture out of a second story window. The man called me and the police. The hospital readmitted her. After ninety days she was discharged. Her self esteem was very low. She couldn't get any work. She wanted to go back to the hospital.

Through the years I always tried to provide her with ordinary supportive family experiences. Often, if not always, things went awry. In 1980, her psychiatrist gave her permission to visit her Aunt Sissy, who lived in upstate New York and was President of Wells College. After six weeks, she left her aunt's home without adequate or protective clothing in 20 degrees below zero weather. She hitchhiked to Syracuse. Lost and alone she called Jerry, our friend who then lived in North Carolina. He was kind enough to drive her across the country and home to me in Austin. Soon after, she asked her psychiatrist to admit her to the hospital. He was discouraged that she had become dependent on the hospital instead of taking responsibility for her behavior. I thought she had recognized her deteriorating condition. The mental health myth, which still had power over me, had me giving her more credit than was probably healthy for her or for me.

On May 9, 1981, Bob and I married. Tarlton and Paul were at my wedding. Gemee had been discharged unexpectedly and without notice the day before to a previous boyfriend now released from the state prison; I did not know where she was. She didn't attend the ceremony.

With a change of presidents in 1981, the National Plan for the Mentally Ill lost all funding. President Reagan attempted to make persons with disabilities, including all persons with chronic mental illness, ineligible for Social Security. Homelessness, homicides and suicides among Gemee's peers increased substantially when many found their existing disability status terminated, and all found it increasingly difficult to establish eligibility for new services and entitlements.

The U.S. Department of Justice entered the R.A.J. lawsuit in Texas and aggressively negotiated the Settlement Agreement of 1981. After many months of negotiating among the parties, a three person panel was appointed to monitor the case. The Panel's Report to the Court in 1982 began to document the failings of the hospital system.

The 1981 Settlement Agreement was put into effect as the Houston police arrested and jailed Gemee for begging on the streets. I had listed her as a missing person, again. Houston's Missing Person Division never checked or cross-listed missing persons with individuals that the police picked up on apparent criminal violations. By jailing Gemee instead of taking her to mental health treatment in the hospital, the police separated her from the general population of individuals with chronic mental illness who were treated in hospitals. They booked her like a criminal; they coerced her, strip-searched her, took mug shots, fingerprinted her and locked her in a cell. Phones in the jail were inaccessible to her, and she couldn't call me. Without treatment, her psychosis naturally escalated. A Houston judge finally decided that she needed hospitalization. He dropped her charges and ordered the police to immediately take her to the hospital for involuntary commitment. I only learned of her whereabouts after the police brought her to Austin State Hospital, and only then because I had frantically and repeatedly called everywhere trying to locate her.

She experienced another unplanned discharge. Off with a man, she overdosed on a medicine that controlled the side effects of her prescribed treatment medication. Her eyes bulged to a bursting point. We waited a long time at her bedside for them to return to a normal size.

Now married to a financially successful man, I no longer had to work and I could focus more time on Gemee's needs. I still believed I could patch together existing laws, funding and services that would support and stabilize her.

By 1983, I gave up on finding laws, policies, services or funding that could wrap around Gemee's cycles of deterioration. Texans with mental illness did not have legal, financial or administrative structures to support them. Their crisis cycles, the voids in aftercare and the deplorable hospital conditions were ignored by the state. Families were relied upon for preventative and aftercare services.

During these two years I looked for families with similar experiences. They were hard to locate, yet I finally found and attended meetings of the Family and Independent Reliance (FAIR) of the Mental Health Association in Texas. This group was part of a statewide family and consumer support system that was nearly invisible. FAIR members supported each other only and did not consider themselves political activists. They intentionally kept anonymous for fear of the stigma of having a mentally ill family member and for fear their loved ones would suffer retaliation from angry hospital staff if they became more assertive in advocating reforms. I located other politically invisible groups for consumers; Dallas, Houston, and San Antonio affiliates of the National Alliance for the Mentally Ill (NAMI). I suggested that our collective advocacy at the Legislature would contribute positively to improving circumstances for our loved one's care and treatment. I was interested in reform and advocacy.

A few individuals joined in begging the State Board of TXMHMR for help with our under staffed and under funded hospitals and community centers. We described the revolving door cycle our loved ones endured, their limited and abusive hospital stays, and the lack of housing options which routed them to uncertified boarding homes and jails. Although we explained the problems we faced, the State Board did not respond. Too few family members and consumers were speaking out to the public and far too many others were silent.

In 1983, Gemee's psychiatrist told her about a new mental health center program of supervised apartments to stabilize hospital dischargees. The only barrier to her participation was that as long as she continued with a private psychiatrist she would be ineligible for the program. Gemee hesitantly terminated her therapy with him to qualify for the apartment program. She started over with a center psychiatrist affiliated with the program. Her schedule included therapy sessions, medication compliance, taking a bus to a work readiness program, housework, shopping and weekly meetings with Mildred, the Project Director, Gemee's direct care workers and me. During her rocky stay, I helped Gemee apply and qualify for Social Security and SSI benefits. Although she had gained weight and was still shaky at the end of three months, she became eligible for a different supervised program. She set her limited employment goals and felt anguished because she could no longer get jobs as she once had.

Under the pressure of maintaining herself with her Social Security and SSI entitlements, she moved to a sub-standard board and care home. After being raped, she moved again to a safer apartment complex. I made two cross town trips per day to ensure that Gemee took her medications and to give her needed emotional support. She worked intermittently across the street from her apartment as a laundry sorter. Gemee was too afraid to get on the bus and make the needed transfer to attend her appointments at the Texas Rehabilitation Commission. She only went when I took her. Her fear was due to her illness and her real life situation. She helped other apartment dwellers who were elderly. She was proud of her tiny efficiency, that she "earned" her entitlements and was improving.

By 1984, I learned that there were approximately five hundred Texans who belonged to NAMI through membership in the Houston and Dallas Affiliates. I became certain I could get the attention of the upcoming Legislature if we became politically visible. Quickly building consensus for a unified and better organization, funding and founding additional urban and rural Affiliates across the state and publishing a State Plan were essential if family members were to have a political impact.

In 1984, following the Review Panel's Third Report on conditions in the state hospitals, the Court entered a finding of non-compliance on the part of the state, specifically citing the lack of staffing, individualized treatment and protection of patients from a high degree of aggressive behavior on the wards throughout the hospital system. Gemee lived through these conditions during her commitment in 1984. The Court also accepted TXMHMR's Rules on Consent to Medication and Standards for the Proper Use of Psychotropic Medications in 1984. These reforms were on paper only, Gemee did not benefit from them. She was dangerously overdosed with Loxitane during her 1984 commitment and forcibly medicated with Thorazine during her commitment in 1989.

The winter of 1983–1984 was unusually bitter cold. In November of 1983, two transients stayed overnight in Gemee's apartment. I saw them as I came to give Gemee her medications. I told them to get out; she and I had worked too hard to stabilize her and get her to this point. She had gained weight and was doing so well. The night before, she and I had enjoyed a ballet performance, and she had a reunion with her former ballet friends. When the men left, Gemee suddenly bolted out the door with them. I waited several hours, but she didn't return. I wished I'd let the transients stay. After 24 hours, I called missing persons and every relevant local and state official for help.

Three months later, Mildred, the sensitive director of the mental health center program where Gemee had been stabilized once before, spotted Gemee under a bridge with two men. Mildred was kind enough to call me. I hired a private detective to help me find her. I drove around Austin daily and continued to pray my rosary novena to Our Lady of Guadalupe. One of my contacts phoned me that the police had arrested Gemee across from the University of Texas. Due to the jail's visitor protocol, I couldn't see her. She had been without treatment for the past three months and would not receive treatment in jail. I knew her psychosis was escalating. After the weekend, the judge dropped her charges and immediately transferred her to the State Hospital. Staff gave her extremely high dosages of Loxitane without attention to the new rules on Consent to Medication and Standards for the Proper Use of Psychotropic Medications.

The staff did not want me to see Gemee for two days because she was so bad off. The question remains with me, "Were they hiding something?" When I finally entered the ward, Gemee wildly leapt in ballet-like steps through the aggressive crowd toward me. She was fifty pounds lighter and her skin had a yellowish tone. We embraced, she rattled in my arms, her teeth chattered, and she told me that she'd lived on ice under the bridge. I was deeply shaken. I felt I needed to protect her, perhaps by becoming her guardian. Her life could no longer be fixed with medication, supports in the community, and prayer alone. Violations of the Settlement Agreement and the absence of state laws, policies, procedures and funding had ravaged her, and I finally realized I had chased a mental health myth for too long.

After Gemee completed a ninety day commitment and had gained weight, the judge committed her for an additional ninety days when he heard her cries of anguish as answers to his questions about her condition. On the way back from her commitment hearing to her ward, she told me she had gone to the hospital beauty shop for a permanent wave. The operator had spilled solution down her neck and back which badly burned her skin. Her skin was raw. I showed staff Gemee's burns. Instead of properly treating her wounds, the staff gave me this response: the Court had found Gemee to be psychotic and only in need of psychiatric treatment, therefore, she was legally competent until a court of law found her incompetent, hence, her burns were her responsibility. Later I took this incident to the Superintendent's office. This administrator made no effort to prevent other burn accidents, nor did the staff on the ward file an injury report. The hospital repeatedly refused her any medical treatment beyond psychiatry, even when physical symptoms, such as this burn, developed during her hospitalizations.

Becoming Gemee's guardian was a difficult, tedious, and time consuming process. I had to go to court to explain her need for my guardianship, accept additional liability and pay the legal expenses involved. The most wrenching requirement was swearing that I believed she would never regain her legal competency. My hope for her recovery had to die for me to become her guardian.

As soon as I was named her guardian, I read her hospital progress notes, itemized many errors of fact, noted extremely high dosages of Loxitane and had her transferred to a private facility where I thought she would be safe. A biopsy confirmed my suspicion that something was terribly wrong; she had induced chemical hepatitis from being overdosed at the hospital, and she would have to be checked regularly for the rest of her life.

After Gemee entered the private facility, I did not have to attend so much to her daily needs. When I had her once a week for day visits, she was delicate. Millions of tears easily flowed, there was no comforting her as she wept in my arms. My son Burney lived until he was eighteen and four months. He passed away in the State School in Corpus Christi in 1982 during a time when Gemee was missing. She missed his funeral. Once she learned of his death in 1984, she was inconsolable. Almost anything set her off; she cried or smiled sadly only to begin crying again.

The R.A.J. lawsuit, the activity of existing mental disability interest groups, multiple interventions of anonymous family members and stories from the media placed pressure upon the Legislature and TXMHMR to change. I helped Gemee and her peers by advocating for an improved public system of mental health care in Texas. Using the time and energy I had previously expended on Gemee's daily needs, I focused on becoming politically visible.

The Mental Health Association invited family members and consumers to a National Institute of Mental Health Community Support

Program in Houston where a friend was elected the Caucus President. I became the "statewide communicator." Austin newspapers had articles about violations of the Settlement Agreement and pending remedies by the legislature.

After the Court's finding non-compliance in 1984, the legislature provided emergency funding to lower the state hospital census, and Lt. Governor Hobby charged the Legislative Oversight Committee to respond with recommendations for the legislature beginning in January 1985. This large committee, in an already tense situation, limited public comment to five minutes at the end of the long days. Patsy, Rachel and Steven Cheyney of San Antonio and I made all the meetings in Austin, and I spoke as the statewide communicator for families and consumers.

A group of us from the Alliances, FAIR and the public founded the Texas Alliance for the Mentally Ill (TEXAMI). Two separate telephone lines on my dining room table rang around-the-clock for information and referrals. I listened and would offer help, and then I would ask the callers to join or form a TEXAMI Affiliate. Bob called our dining room "world headquarters."

In February 1985, my mother died. The doctors said she had Alzheimer's. As I looked through my mother's albums, I found many letters written by my father to my mother addressed to a private hospital. As my father placed me with different families during my childhood, I was always told that my mother was on vacation or in the hospital. I reconsidered her erratic, violent, horrid behavior and questioned whether she had been mentally ill. When one of my three remaining siblings refused to consent to contributing my mother's brain to research, I never felt so strongly about shedding anonymity. Scientific fact about our mother's brain could have provided valuable information for all of us. Sadly, I came from a well-educated middle-class family that still hid from the shame of mental illness.

In March 1985, I testified in Federal Court for the plaintiffs on the lack of post-hospitalization aftercare. I also testified before the Texas Legislature on the need to fund quality hospital and community care. The Court entered a finding that the State was providing inadequate aftercare for hospital patients. The Legislature granted more funding to lower the hospital census. TXMHMR created an incentive funding process designed to foster rapid development of support services for discharged hospital patients. Mental health centers developed crisis centers and supervised apartments across the state. New options for aftercare blossomed and the hospital census decreased. Staff to patient ratios were improved to a point acceptable to the Court.

That spring Gemee grew thinner, cried torrents and ran away. After ten days, the staff of the private facility found and readmitted her. That summer we attended Rhonda's wedding. I ached over Gemee's many losses and realized she probably would never have her own wedding. I squarely faced that I had to accept a standard for her different from an average mother's expectations for her daughter's happiness. Her tears were steady and many.

In 1986, her psychiatrist, Dr. Day, died. Gemee refused her medication and the staff of the private facility did not honor her right to refuse. They forced her to take the medication. She ran away once again, but within an hour called me, sobbing, to help her. I confronted the staff. They agreed not to force her medications again and to call me if she refused. Days later she ran off again and called me to help her.

Meanwhile, TEXAMI members went to Waco to speak to the Chair of the State Board of TXMHMR. I went with Houston Affiliate members to meet with their Board Representative. We asked for larger budgets for staffing of hospitals and community centers. The TEXAMI Executive Committee also met regularly to influence a legislative committee which made TXMHMR reauthorization recommendations to the upcoming Legislature in January 1987.

From 1984 through 1987, I was founding affiliates, making TEXAMI politically visible and providing additional private Art Therapy for Gemee. Moe, her Art Therapist, provided political visibility for schizophrenia in the Rotunda of the State Capitol in 1987. She displayed Gemee's paintings with the written descriptions Gemee had prepared for each one. Observers keenly noted how Gemee's various descriptions delineated her oncoming states of disintegration, crisis, and recovery from active episodes of schizophrenia. Cycles of schizophrenia were clear in her paintings and writing even to those unfamiliar with the ravages of this illness.

TEXAMI had grown from four to thirty-three Affiliates with a mailing list of 3,000 and had a savvy political platform. After consulting with knowledgeable people, I began a campaign of "$40 million more" when giving testimony and talking to legislators. This increase was desperately needed for community services. The TXMHMR

Board refused to ask for more money. In March, I organized a press conference in the Lt. Governor's Press Room for the director of Whisper Oaks Board and Care Home from Palestine. TXMHMR planned to cut her funds for community beds. She described the inevitable and impending consequences of funding cuts on her clients who had been discharged to her care by Rusk State Hospital. In thirty days her clients would be on the streets. After the press conference, the R.A.J. Court Monitor and TXMHMR legal staff went to Whisper Oaks on a fact finding expedition. The press followed and the media focused on the issues which concerned us, especially the badly needed community services. This issue gained momentum.

"$40 Million More" caught on. At an Appropriation Committee Hearing, the Commissioner of TXMHMR did a turnaround and asked for $158 million increase in his budget. In my testimony, I continued to plug "$40 Million More." An Appropriation Committee Legislator, asked the R.A.J. Court Monitor if a $40 million increase would get the state out of the lawsuit. The Court Monitor answered that the amount in and of itself would not resolve the lawsuit, but it would go a long way to help. I felt we were at a turning point: we were going to get what we asked for.

Progress was being made for system improvements even while horrible backslides occurred. I experienced the same pattern with Gemee. By the fall of 1987, Gemee was deteriorating even further at the private facility. I took her to another private psychiatrist for an evaluation. This physician said that Gemee was "hard core" and unlikely to improve at all, if ever. She advised me to closely work with a doctor in either the public or private system. I had to make a choice. I was concerned that the private facility would continue to forcibly medicate her even though they promised they would not. According to Gemee's progress notes, she frothed at the mouth, rolled her eyes back, resisted force and lost five pounds during one of these ordeals.

When Gemee went into crisis again, I asked for her transfer to the Acute Care Unit (ACU) at the State Hospital. The R.A.J. Monitor's long battle had focused much attention upon improving hospital staffing and substantial gains were occurring. Staff now welcomed Gemee and the fact that she had a guardian. While the ACU was short on staff, they tended to Gemee's dental and other physical needs. Her art therapist was able to continue her work with Gemee on the hospital grounds, and staff included Gemee and me as a part of her Treatment Team.

Again Gemee refused medications. Staff, Tarlton, Paul, a family friend, and I explained the benefits of her medications on our visits which were occurring at least twice a day. One evening, she surprised me and took her medications.

Having her on the ACU, where several people had recently killed themselves, was alarming. After my continuous complaints, I learned that ACU staff were shuffled to other units to handle staff shortages. It was tragic that the ACU was short staffed. This was where patients were admitted in deep psychosis, needed emergency care and were often suicidal. I told her doctor that Gemee needed to be in a unit with adequate staffing. If I had not been politically aware, I would not have recognized the staff-patient ratio issue nor known how to address Gemee's precarious situation in December.

Staff transferred Gemee to the Extended Care Unit (ECU). While the ECU had adequate staffing for "hopeless patients," there was little programming. Other units at least had "Psychosocial Programs." I worked with the new Superintendent, Kenny Dudley, to add "Social Learning" to the ECU.

The R.A.J. Monitor worked to have the heating, cooling and water fountains function properly. Although the ECU staff did not allow day passes, we could walk together around the beautifully wooded hospital grounds. Nature's asylum and Mass held at the hospital on Sundays were our solace. Gemee was very thin, often in tears and easily frightened. She did not want to leave the grounds. Too often she was put in a quiet room or a seclusion room for not behaving. She did not understand the criteria for being released from confinement; staff did not know how to relate to her during their fifteen minute check points. Her paranoia and their inability to communicate exacerbated and prolonged her confinement. I worked with staff who needed guidance, training and nurturing. Finally they grasped how to help her learn how to gain release from seclusion.

A new TXMHMR Commissioner of Mental Health, Dennis Jones, arrived in Texas in 1988. He defined hospital patients as "Consumers of Mental Health Services." He focused on their needs and was eager to have input from consumer, family, and advocacy organizations. The new Commissioner had Masters Degrees in both Social Work

44   State Hospital Reform: Why Was It So Hard to Accomplish?

and Business. He eventually implemented a state-wide hospital system measured by objective data to ensure quality professional standards, and he gradually added staff to monitor Continuous Quality Improvements (CQI). For the next six years, he spoke to legislators in business terms of quality improvement, asked for increased funding and diverted their attention from the R.A.J. lawsuit. The Court Monitor wrote more reports that included statistical findings about aftercare needs and the parties struggled for a resolution to the issues of the lawsuit.

Gemee found a boyfriend who was her age. She enjoyed Billy until he was suddenly transferred. While their relationship lasted, I had a glimmer of their joy and fun. I saw them kissing between the curtains and the glass wall as I approached the ECU building. No one on the ward could see them; they found a moment of privacy on the crowded floor.

After Billy's transfer, Gemee had very bad days. She was transferred to the Intensive Care Unit (ICU), a behavioral program for aggressive patients who assaulted staff and other patients. Gemee was confused, fearful and badly bruised by other patients there. In order to return to the ECU she had to behave well for five successive days, documented by staff at fifteen minute intervals of observation. The unit rule on the ICU which was different than the ECU was that any altercation during any fifteen minute period resulted in her having to start over. Paul, Tarlton, a family friend, and I worked with her to build half and full days of good behavior; after three weeks she completed one four day stretch before having to start over. Rational consequences were difficult for Gemee to understand and act upon when she was psychotic. It was also difficult to tell whether her injuries were always real. She cried and complained of being with criminals. She did not comprehend our analyzing her fifteen minute progress record to help her continue improving. She was oblivious to the requirements for release and was only motivated by fear. We were all afraid for her, and we rotated two of us at a time visiting her twice daily for fifteen minutes, which was the maximum allowed. In her sixth week, she completed the required five days of appropriate behavior.

Back on the ECU, she had a more supportive physical environment. Newly placed over-stuffed chairs and sofas were in clusters around the unit, pictures were hung and the TV was in a section rather than blaring all over the room. Efforts were clearly being made to make the unit more livable and comfortable. Still, temperatures erratically fluctuated from the faulty heating and cooling system.

She faced danger again when a male patient, transferred from the maximum security hospital, raped two women and tried to rape her in the toilet/shower area. After this transgression, staff returned the man to his former hospital and locked the restroom area. Patients had to ask for access to the restrooms to use them. Understaffing was still a problem and the institutional quality of the unit returned. Hard-won progress for patients rights eroded. Sexual assaults continued despite staff monitoring.

In 1989, Gemee once more refused medications and for three weeks she deteriorated badly. The doctor wanted to force medicate her and asked my permission as her guardian. I did not want to repeat the experience of the forced medication she endured in the private facility. He agreed to wait until I arrived to see if Gemee would be willing to take her medication while I was with her. The doctor and Gemee were both smiling when I arrived. She had taken a high dose of Thorazine after the doctor had taken advantage of her current delusion of being a doctor; he had told her to choose whatever medication and reminded her that the dosage had to be high and regular. She had agreed. This was a manipulative trick, and while effective, I question its appropriateness.

Within a short time Gemee was more coherent. Her tears stopped. She progressed to the point that the staff planned to transfer her to the Transitional Living Unit (TLU). As she was about to take this step forward, she inexplicably developed a dangerously high fever and was transferred to Brackenridge Hospital where her doctor performed exploratory surgery. He recommended a hysterectomy. She was badly infected and torn up. I consented on the condition that he not allow her to go into psychosis. He provided her with one-on-one staffing. She remained coherent and determinedly walked in physical pain the day after surgery. Focused on recovery, she ate and moved around with vigor. Her tears stopped; her ready smile and focus returned. She re-entered the ECU. I thanked God for her survival and a "New Day."

These years of mistreatment including staff setting unrealistic goals; staff neglecting her medical, dental and psychiatric treatment to a point where her mistreatment resulted in a chemical hepatitis; her living in wards where she was unprotected, beaten up, burned, almost raped, secluded beyond need, forcibly medicated; and repeated discharges without plans and procedures to enter the community were behind her. She would learn to dream differently and to be proud of her gradual improvement.

In the fall of 1989, the ECU staff was eager to begin the Social Learning program. At that time, they transferred Gemee from the ECU to the TLU. She steadily gained confidence, earned passes, left the grounds, spent the night with me and spent half days at her prospective personal care home. In the spring of 1990, the Social Learning program began on the ECU as Gemee was successfully discharged from the TLU to Crest Oak, an Austin-Travis County Mental Health and Mental Retardation Center (ATCMHMR) personal care home where she improved.

Step-by-baby-step, Gemee progressed in the ATCMHMR Work Readiness Program. She worked in the Thrift Shop and earned her first dollars in a decade; eventually she ran the cash register. Proudly and happily, she bought a pair of shoes and a purse with her first paycheck.

In 1991, the Court Monitor and the TXMHMR found common ground. The R.A.J./ Quality System's Oversight (QSO) proposal was developed as a means of resolving continuing problems in the hospitals. The QSO process required the involvement of consumers and their advocates.

I became a QSO team consultant and was on a team with other family members, consumers, psychiatrists and psychologists. Families and consumers used Patients Rights Instruments which measured rights protections on the hospital wards.

Gemee has lived a life far from the promise she once held as a girl who was capable of dancing professionally. She has a heavy smoker's cough, carries many excess pounds for her 5'3" frame, and has chemical hepatitis and recurring delusions.

I am pleased to say she has steadily kept a two hour a day janitorial job since 1993 and has maintained her mental gains through three apartment moves. She now lives alone, across the street from the ATCMHMR Center in apartments where sixteen other consumers live. She attends the committee and board meetings, the Center's programs, has a case manager, and plans to learn to use a computer and take more art classes.

She has a bountiful and loving nature which has not been destroyed. She is hopeful and daydreams of ways to make herself happy. In 1996, she suggested having a belated Mother's Day luncheon with Louise, Paul and me. Louise is a loyal, dependable and generous woman who had two sons with mental illness. During the eighties, one committed suicide and the other was killed on his bicycle. She has been by my side in advocacy and been a friend to Gemee ever since we met her in 1983.

At our luncheon, Gemee gave Louise and me a long stemmed, thornless red rose. The waiter took our group picture. We recalled how the system was when we met and all the progress made since. We acknowledged that our hospital reforms are still very fragile. Afterward, as we stood outside talking, Gemee breathed in deeply, arched her back and stepped into a ballet position. She twirled her strong, gracefully muscled legs from first through fifth positions.

At moments like this, I ask myself, "Does the family of each consumer have to become politically active to see their children's heart set free? — to keep the mental health system vigilant?" My answer is emphatically, "YES!" We must keep on in order for our children's tears to ever be turned into dancing. For this "New Day," we must continue strengthening the reforms and making gradual gains like Gemee makes in her daily life. I pray to live to see her mental illness burn off with age and to feel certain that the R.A.J. reforms are solidified beyond any possibility of erosion.

Timeline

	History	Gemee	U.S. Mental Health Events	R.A.J. Lawuit
1957		Gemee is born.		
1960	Kennedy elected.	Her sister is born. Gemee using poetic language: "The sun is melting out."	Martin Birnbaum writing in the American Bar Assn Journal defines right to treatment.	
1963	Kennedy assasinated.	Her brother is born.	Community Mental Health Centers Construction Act.	
1964	President Johnson' Omnibus Civil Rights Bill enacted.	Family moves back to Texas. Brother diagnosed with mental retardation.		
1965	Medicare medical coverage under Social Security initiated.	Parents divorce. Gemee telling imaginative stories in grade school.		
1967		Gemee wins awards in grade school science fair, and at camp.	Thomas Szasz publishes influential article "The Myth of Mental Illness."	
1968	Nixon elected.	Her stepbrother is born. She wins a ballet talent show.	National Alliance for the Mentally Ill is founded.	
1970		Complicated custody battle. Gemee becomes unreachable. "Ran away from headaches." Family referred to psychologist.	Wyatt v. Stickney, first mental health institutional reform lawsuit filed in Alabama.	
1974	Nixon resigns and Gerald Ford becomes president.	Gemee joins Austin Ballet Company. First hospitalization on Adolescent Unit.		R.A.J. lawsuit filed.
1975	The VietNam war ends as Saigon falls. "One Flew Over The Cuckoo's Nest" wins Academy Award as Best Picture.	Gemee begins cycles of runaways, hospitalizations, and periods of living on the street or in jail.	O'Connor v. Donaldson, patient ordered dismissed from mental hospital because his right to treatment has been violated.	

	History	Gemee	U.S. Mental Health Events	R.A.J. Lawsuit
1976	Carter elected president. U.S. celebrates its 200th birthday.	Gemee is jailed for panhandling. Hospitalized for suicidal behavior. Run aways. Unplanned pregnancy. Additional hospitalizations; hospital denies responsibility for injuries.		
1978			Congress passes and funds national plan for chronically mentally ill, but newly elected president voids funding Rogers v. Okin ruling on right to refuse medication.	Efforts to settle the R.A.J. suit fall through. U.S. Department of Justice enters the case and aggressively presses for a settlement.
1981	Sandra Day O'Connor confirmed as first woman Supreme Court Justice. Hinkley shoots President Reagan.	Gemee's mother remarries. Gemee hospitalized again; is then discharged to a known predator. Overdoses.	Sylvia Frumkin story appears in the New Yorker as "Is There No Place On Earth For Me?" Rennie v. Klein ruling on right to refuse medication.	First R.A.J. settlement.
1982	Equal Rights Amendment fails to receive ratification by states.	Gemee living in an apartment with mother coming daily to give medication. Brother dies in state school for the retarded.	Youngberg v. Romeo limits the definition of right to treatment, by making "professional judgment" the standard for care.	R.A.J. Review Panel appointed by the Federal Court. Implementation phase begin.
1983		Gemee runs away with predators; jailed again for panhandling; hospitalized again. Mother becomes legal guardian.	E. Fuller Torrey publishes *Surviving Schizophrenia: A Family Manual.*	Standards developed for the proper use of psychotropic medication.
1984	Ronald Regan reelected.	Gemee runs away from a private hospital; is readmitted. Mother founds the Texas Alliance for the Mentally Ill (TEXAMI).		Compliance court hearing finds state noncompliance on three issues; accepts medication rules. Legislature appropriates emergency funds to implement staff ratios.
1985		Gemee's grandmother dies. Gemee's art is shown in the state capitol rotunda.		$35.50 Program hearing on adequacy of community care.

	History	Gemee	U.S. Mental Health Events	R.A.J. Lawuit
1986	William Rehnquist confirmed as Chief Justice of the U.S. Supreme Court. Space shuttle *Challenger* explosion.	Gemee's private psychiatrist who had worked with her for 6 years dies.	E.F. Torry & S.M. Wolfe publish *Care of the Seriously Mentally Ill* which for the first time offers comprehensive ratings of the quality of each state's programs for the mentally ill.	Adequate community aftercare defined.
1987		Private hospital did not honor Gemee's right to refuse medication.	Lelsz v. Kavanagh ruling closes the door to federal court intervention in community mental health aftercare. Gabbard & Gabbard publish *Psychiatry and the Cinema* showing the consistenty distorted, negative depiction of psychiatry in U.S. films.	U.S. Justice Department withdraws from the R.A.J. case stating it was unable to support the Court and the Monitor with respect to community aftercare.
1988	George Bush elected.	A consultant tells Gemee's mother to act as advocate and choose either public or private system for care. Transfers Gemee back to ASH hoping R.A.J. reforms had led to improvements, and becomes member of treatment team. Gemee consents to medication and experiences several successes. Is transferred to Extended Care, and is sexually assulted on unit; too psychotic to meet 15 minute criteria of calm. Relatives and friends sit with her nearly continuously.		TXMHMR appoints new commissioner. R.A.J. structure changes from Review Panel to Monitor.

May Our Tears Be Turned into Dancing 51

	History	Gemee	U.S. Mental Health Events	R.A.J. Lawuit
1989	Exxon Valdez oil spill in Alaska. Oliver North convicted in Iran-Contra related trial.	Gemee is transferred to Transitional Living Program at ASH. Has emergency hysterectomy.		Recognizing improvements in use of meds, adequate staffing JCAHO accreditation, and life safety code factors, the court dismisses those issues.
1990	Americans With Disabilities Act signed by President Bush. Justice Brennan retires and David Souter is nominated to replace him.	Following her 14th and last hospitalization, Gemee is moved to community center personal care home.		Community aftercare report disputed.
1991	U.S. led coalition defeats Iraq in Gulf War.	Her friend is murdered in the personal care home.		14th Report to the Court results in negotiation of a new Settlement Agreement.
1992	Clinton-Gore ticket wins presidential election.			New Settlement Agreement yields development of QSO process.
1993	Ruth Bader Ginsburg sworn in as 2nd woman Supreme Court Justice.	Gemee moves to apartment program, works at a sheltered workshop and at Goodwill. Moves to Section 8 housing.		Hospitals begin to comply with eight specified requirements
1994	President Clinton's efforts to enact a comprehensive health-care reform bill falter as the Senate Majority Leader withdraws support for its passage.			First state hospitals is released from the suit after achieving full compliance.
1997				Court issues final ruling closing the R.A.J. case.

Chapter 3

History of Mental Health Legal Issues

David Pharis

As an outgrowth of the Civil Rights movement in the late 1960's, federal courts became involved in protecting the constitutional rights of persons in state and federal mental health, mental retardation, and correctional institutions. The constitutional issues for mental health and mental retardation patients were primarily covered by interpretations of the Fourteenth and Eighth Amendments. Incarceration in an institution without the provision of treatment was considered to be incarceration without protection of the individual's due process rights and also a form of cruel and unusual punishment.

Several new legal concepts were established through mental health litigation during the 1970's. Landmark cases established the right to treatment, the right to treatment in the least restrictive environment, the right to be protected from harm, the recognition of a number of patient rights which should be maintained during hospitalization, and the right to consent to or refuse treatment. These requirements became definitions of constitutional protections. Case law was often established in individual cases and precedents were incorporated in class action lawsuits. A settlement agreement in such a class action lawsuit usually defined how the state agency was to provide services. Some court cases were aimed at improving the living and treatment conditions within facilities. Other cases had the philosophical orientation that treatment services should be provided in community based programs with deinstitutionalization as a goal.

The legal issues which give the federal court jurisdiction over the operation of state mental hospitals were defined in the 1960's and the 1970's.[1] In their recent book, *Madness in the Streets: How Psychiatry*

---

1. McPheeters, H. L. *Implementing Standards to Assure the Rights of Mental Patients*, (Summary) Proceedings of Symposium, Atlanta, Georgia, June 1–3, 1977 (DHHS Publication No. ADM 80-860). Rockville, Md., National Institute of Health, 1980.

and the Law Abandon the Mentally Ill, Isaac and Armat specifically argue that the emergence of the Mental Health Bar represented an acceptance of the ideas of anti-psychiatrists, R.D.Laing and Thomas Szasz.[2] In their own way both Laing and Szasz argued that there was no such thing as mental illness.[3][4][5] Laing held a clinical position which argued that the behaviors characterized as mental illness by the rest of society were often the reactions of the sane individual to the requirements of an insane world. Szasz did not debate the clinical realities of the existence of mental illness, but rather argued the civil libertarian position that placing people in institutions is a means by which society controls its members. Isaac and Armat argue that the civil libertarians of the Mental Health Bar opposed involuntary commitment from the position that whether mental illness exists or not, people should not be locked up for reasons other than those determined through due process proceedings.

In Rouse v. Cameron, the court addressed the concept of the right to treatment previously articulated by Morton Birnbaum in an American Bar Association Journal article.[6][7] The court granted the plaintiff's petition that he be released after three years of involuntary commitment on the grounds that he had received no psychiatric treatment. Justice Bazelon wrote the opinion which established the first determination of a constitutional right to treatment. The court stated: "Absence of treatment might draw in to question the constitutionality of this mandatory commitment section.... It has also been suggested that failure to supply treatment may violate the equal protection clause. Indefinite confinement without treatment of one who has been found not criminally responsible may be so inhumane as to be cruel and unusual punishment."[8] This quote, however, reflects a question of the court rather than the establishment of a legal princi-

---

2. Isaac, Rael Jean, and Armat, Virginia C., *Madness in the Streets*, New York, The Free Press, 1980, pp. 17–65.

3. Laing, R.D., *The Politics of Experience*, New York, Ballantine, 1967.

4. Laing, R.D., *The Divided Self*, New York, Pantheon; 1969.

5. Szasz, Thomas, "The Myth of Mental Illness," in Thomas Scheff, ed., *Mental Illness and Social Process*, New York, Harper and Row, 1967.

6. Rouse v. Cameron, 373 F. 2d [dc cir. 1966].

7. Birnbaum, Morton; "The Right to Treatment," *American Bar Association Journal*, 46, 1960, pp. 490–503.

8. Rouse v. Cameron, 373. 2d(a) 453 [dc cir. 1966].

pal. The decision was based upon reversal of the lower court decision on statutory rather than constitutional grounds.

The first application of the right to treatment concept in a class action lawsuit appeared in the filing of Wyatt v. Stickney in 1970.[9] The Plaintiffs, both staff and patients of Alabama's Bryce Hospital, sought the rehiring of the employees fired due to state budget reductions and the closing of hospital admissions to insure continued care of patients. The suit alleged that the firing of the employees placed patients at risk by exposing them to inadequate treatment. The Federal District Court concluded that patient treatment did not meet any minimal standards of treatment of the mentally ill. In 1971, the Court amended the case to include mentally retarded patients from two state schools. Initially the hospital and the two schools were given six months to improve care.

Six months later U.S. District Judge Johnson determined that treatment was inadequate in three areas: humane, psychological, and physical environment; qualified staff in sufficient numbers to administer adequate treatment; and individualized treatment plans. The American Association of Mental Deficiency, the American Psychological Association, the American Orthopsychiatric Association, and the American Civil Liberties Union all entered this case as amici curiae. These organizations recommended standards to the court for the provision of adequate treatment. The order and decree of April 13, 1972 established standards covering all aspects of treatment in the facilities.[10] These standards were extremely prescriptive, defining the numbers and qualifications of staff and the details of patients rights. Specific environmental requirements such as the size of day rooms, the number of toilets per patient, and adequate temperature ranges were established. The Court also specified the content of patient records and treatment plans.

The state of Alabama immediately appealed the Federal District Court's ruling. Although the court order was upheld, the attempts at implementation of such a specific court order proved to be inordinately costly. It also became apparent that the facilities were unable to hire all of the required staff.

---

9. Wyatt v. Stickney, CA 3195-N (M.D. Ala. 1971).
10. Wyatt v. Stickney, CA 3195-N (M.D. Ala. 1972).

The right to liberty, as distinguished from the right to treatment, was determined by the U.S. Supreme Court in the O'Connor v. Donaldson decision in 1975. Hospitalized against his will for 14 years, Kenneth Donaldson had repeatedly refused treatment. The court determined that patients "who are not dangerous to themselves or others, are receiving only custodial care and are capable of surviving safely and freely or with the help of family or friends" should not be hospitalized against their will.[11] The O'Connor v. Donaldson ruling further clarified the judicial basis for the right to treatment defined in earlier cases.

Since involuntarily committed patients are hospitalized as a protection from harm and the hospital must provide treatment it seems unusual that there could be a legal argument that such a patient has the right to refuse treatment. Such arguments, however, have been made and two precedent setting court cases have established different models for permitting such patients to refuse medication. Rennie v. Klein, a New Jersey case, places decision making about the medical necessity and appropriateness of the treatment in the hands of the medical professional.[12] Rogers v. Okin, a Massachusetts case, establishes due process procedures through court review to determine the patient's competency to make the consent decision.[13] Decided at approximately the same time, each case went in a different direction in considering such issues as the determination of competency to make informed consent. However, both cases recognize the existence of psychiatric emergencies and permit forced medication during such an emergency.

Both of these decision-making models have advocates and critics. Physicians often support the administrative model of Rennie v. Klein because it maintains the professional judgment of physicians and retains decision making within the sphere of clinical practice. Civil libertarian attorneys are usually critical of this model and support the due process determination of competency as the proper form of determining this issue.

In 1980, the United States Congress enacted the Civil Rights of Institutionalized Persons Act (CRIPA).[14] The purpose of this act was to

---

11. O'Connor v. Donaldson, 422 U.S. 1975.
12. Rennie v. Klein, 720 F. 2d (3rd Cir. 1983).
13. Rogers v. Okin, 634 F. 2d 650 (1st Cir. 1980).
14. CRIPA, 42 U.S.C.–1997 J.

authorize the United State Department of Justice to litigate against states to protect the constitutional rights of the institutionalized. The legislation required that complaints must identify grievous patterns of practice rather than isolated incidents. When situations of violations of CRIPA are discovered by the Justice Department, the Justice Department must attempt voluntary settlement which includes corrective measures of the pattern of practice prior to litigation of the case. The United States Department of Justice has been criticized since 1980 for the manner in which it has implemented CRIPA. Protection and advocacy agencies and other mental health advocates have maintained that there has been less than enthusiastic enforcement. CRIPA, however, does represent one level of federal intervention in state facilities for the purpose of providing constitutional protections.

The most recent court decision which affected the rights of patients in institutions was the 1982 Supreme Court ruling in Youngberg v. Romeo. That ruling narrowed and restricted the interpretations of the standard of right to treatment which had been partially established through the earlier cases.[15] The Plaintiffs argued that the patient, an individual from Pennhurst State School, had been placed in physical restraints for long periods without receiving alternative forms of habilitation or treatment. The court concluded that an individual in a state institution did not have an absolute right to treatment but rather should be protected from harm, should not be caused to deteriorate in condition, and should be subject to treatment based on the judgment of a qualified professional. As this case involved a mentally retarded patient and a state school, it could be argued that it does not apply to the mentally ill in state hospitals. However, the Romeo standards of protection from harm and the presumed validity of professional judgments have become the standards for interpreting the level of care required in state institutions used by the U.S. Department of Justice in their management of litigation.

The cases reviewed above present the legal issues which are now the basis for mental health case law concerning hospitalized individuals. This case law is partial in nature. Some of the rights are not fully established and there can be questions about the absolute nature of such rights.

---

15. Youngberg v. Romeo, 457 U.S. 307 (1982)

58   State Hospital Reform: Why Was It So Hard to Accomplish?

Prior to the Supreme Court's findings in Youngberg v. Romeo it appeared as if the liberal interpretations of the rights of the mentally ill and mentally retarded in institutions, which were established during the 1970's, would continue. The findings in Youngberg v. Romeo marked the move to legal conservatism which has continued to the present.[16] [17] Youngberg v. Romeo represented a conservative limitation of the rights of the disabled in institutions. The actions of the Civil Rights Division of the United States Department of Justice as they implemented CRIPA represented an administrative response to the legal interpretation expressed by the Romeo findings. These legal and administrative actions reflected the movement towards social conservatism of the Reagan and Bush administrations.

In his book, *The Hollow Hope*, Rosenberg discusses the role of the court in such cases. The turn from liberal to more conservative interpretations of the law illustrates three main areas of conflict: the nature of the rights protected by the constitution, states' rights versus federation, and the involvement of federal courts as activists. There is also the question of what is the role, if any, of federal courts in producing significant social reform. The "dynamic court" view sees courts as powerful vigorous proponents of change. The "constrained court" view limits the activism of the court and emphasizes that the concern of the court should be the interpretation of the law rather than the effects of the law.[18] The polarity between the positions of dynamic court view versus a constrained court view are similar to the polarity between a liberal interpretation of legal rights versus a limited interpretation.

The success of social reform litigation in the last 40 years promoted the courts as an appropriate means for promoting social change. The logic appeared to be that litigation would define rights as protected by constitutional, federal, or state laws, and courts then would order remedies. The definitions of the rights of the mentally ill obtained in the 1970's emerged through this process. The subsequent

---

16. Perlin, Michael L., *Law and the Delivery of Mental Health Services in the Community*, American Journal of Orthopsychiatry, 64(2), April 1994.

17. La Fond, John Q., "Law and the Delivery of Involuntary Mental Health Services," *American Journal of Orthopsychiatry*, 64(2), April 1994.

18. Rosenberg, Gerald N., *The Hollow Hope*, Chicago, The University of Chicago, 1991, pp. 9–36.

restriction of these legal interpretations of rights to some extent reflected a shift toward belief in a "constrained court."

In a discussion of the constrained court view versus the dynamic court view, Rosenberg presents four conditions necessary for a dynamic court to effectively produce social change and three arguments by the proponents of the constrained role of the court.[19] These constraints and conditions are not diametrically opposed to each other but rather appear to illustrate some of the complexities of litigation and the process of change. The constraints on the courts ordering social reform are threefold. Legal rights are not unlimited but are defined by the constitution and by federal and state statute. There are definite procedures in place which limit how rights are defined and determined. The judiciary lacks the necessary independence from the other branches of government to produce significant social reform. Since judges are often appointed politically, they are often dependant upon those who appointed them and lack the political constituency of an elected official. Court decisions, therefore, may not be supported by public opinion. The judiciary lacks the power of implementation. Although the judiciary can determine that a state needs to improve its mental health care, it does not directly have the authority to appropriate the funds or administer the agency in a way that assures implementation will take place. The conditions needed for the ready implementation of court-ordered mandates include specific incentives which could motivate the administrators of the mental health agency to make improvements. Courts may effectively produce important social change if the legislature supports the reforms, or when agency administrators use the court as a lever for requesting funds from the legislature.[20]

The four conditions for successful court reform presuppose the willing participation of the actors. The constraints against successful court reform are identified as lack of tools, resources, and authority to make these actors cooperate. The court certainly does not have absolute authority to ensure that their decisions are carried out. It only has authority over the specific Parties to the specific case. Although

---

19. Ibid. pp. 33–35.
20. Ibid. pp. 33–35.

the courts have the authority to hold Defendants in contempt of court or to levy fines or establish such remedies as placement of an agency into receivership, courts are often reluctant to take such action because these actions would certainly be appealed and could produce a constitutional crisis regarding the authority of the different branches of government.

Granted the constraints that the court has on ensuring implementation of its orders, the court is dependant upon the good faith efforts of the Parties to the case. Mechanisms available to the court to ensure such good faith include monitoring implementation efforts, negotiation between the Parties, judicial court orders for actions, judicial reviews, and the power to order some ultimate legal consequences for noncompliance with court orders.

Judge David Bazelon, a federal district judge who wrote the landmark decision in Rouse v. Cameron, discusses the difficulties inherent in a federal court becoming involved in ordering technical reforms in the area of psychiatry. His comments illustrate the concerns expressed by the three constraints to court-ordered reform identified by Rosenberg. Judge Bazelon writes: "Courts are not as competent as hospitals to make treatment decisions. The evaluation of standards of adequacy and suitability may be next to impossible in the present state of psychiatry where 'treatment' means different things to different psychiatrists. No matter how much compulsive treatment is afforded, compulsory hospitalization is itself generally based on ill conceded standards and goals and ought to be reformed radically or discontinued all together. The real problem is one of inadequate resources, which the courts are helpless to remedy — the question posed is one for the legislature and is a basic policy judgment involving overall priorities in the allocation of scarce resources."[21]

This chapter discuses relevant court cases which have established the direction of mental health law concerning hospitalized individuals. Case law is partial in nature and the direction of decisions has changed within the last 30 years. Early decisions were liberal to the extent that they established rights of patients in institutions and established the right to be treated without harm and to receive a level of active treatment. This case law seemed to establish government's responsibility towards disabled institutionalized individuals. Later

---

21. Bazelon, D., in D. Burris (ed.), *The Right to Treatment,* New York, 1969.

court decisions limited government's responsibilities to provide such services.

The constraints upon litigation achieving social reform and the conditions within which litigation can be expected to achieve social reform will be discussed throughout this book. The steps of the legal adversarial process, which include negotiated agreement, monitoring, judicial reviews, and further negotiations will be examined.

Chapter 4

The History of the R.A.J.
Lawsuit in Texas

David Pharis

The class action lawsuit, R.A.J. v. TXMHMR Commissioner filed against the Texas Department of Mental Health and Mental Retardation (TXMHMR) was intended to reform the state's eight state psychiatric hospitals. "R.A.J." are the initials of the lead plaintiff's name. In many chapter references the case name will be R.A.J. v. Miller, R.A.J. v. Jones, or R.A.J. v. Gilbert. These various names refer to the Commissioner at the time. The parents of patients in several of the hospitals filed the case in the United States District Court in 1974. Judge Barefoot Sanders presided over this case from 1979 through its conclusion in 1997.

Although the suit was filed in 1974, no movement occurred until reviews of the hospitals were conducted in 1980 by experts representing the Civil Rights Division of the United States Department of Justice which had entered the case as amicus curiae. At this point the Plaintiffs, Defendants, and Amicus Curiae negotiated a Settlement Agreement aimed at alleviating the conditions identified in the experts' reports.

The original complaint in the R.A.J. litigation alleged that patients' constitutional rights were being violated due to lack of active treatment, the misuse of psychotropic medications, and unsafe conditions.

According to the Plaintiffs' 1980 Amended Complaint, the named Plaintiffs included:[1]

---

1. R.A.J. v. Kavanagh, Plaintiffs' Amended Complaint, 1980.

- A thirty-one-year-old mentally retarded man who was placed in a hospital in a small room often without a bed, chair, or access to a toilet. He remained in the room without treatment, meaningful exercise, or any opportunity to acquire new skills.

- A sixty-five-year-old woman who lived in an overcrowded dormitory which deprived her of all privacy. She received inappropriate and unnecessary dosages of medication and electroshock therapy. Although she was diagnosed as having involuntary movements, psychotropic medications were not reduced.

- A twelve-year-old non-psychotic emotionally disturbed girl who was placed on a multiple disabilities unit with multiply handicapped, mentally retarded, and psychotic individuals. According to the Plaintiffs, she did not need hospitalization.

- A forty-eight-year-old man who was rehospitalized due to his refusing medications. Medication refusal was not dealt with as a treatment issue and there were other indications of inadequate aftercare planning.

- A twenty-year-old mentally retarded man who was primarily managed through the use of extensive seclusion. At one point he remained in seclusion for approximately a five-month period. He may have been subjected to serious physical abuse and injury requiring some medical treatment.

- A forty-eight-year-old woman who had many admissions to the hospital. She received inappropriate and unnecessary dosages of psychotropic medication and did not receive rehabilitative treatment aimed at enabling her to return to independent community living.

- A eighty-eight-year-old woman who was living on the second floor of an overcrowded building which reeked of urine and was not equipped with an elevator. This person, who was not considered by Plaintiffs to require hospitalization, was kept on a locked ward, denied basic privacy, subjected to assault by other patients and denied the opportunity to have personal possessions.

- A thirty-one-year-old man who was on the maximum security unit for alleged verbally threatening behavior but was receiving no program to decrease this problem behavior.

The Settlement Agreement negotiated in 1981 specified the following requirements:[2]

- protection of patients rights,

- provision of individualized treatment,

- adequate staffing to provide thirty hours of appropriate pro gramming to patients,

- renovation of buildings to meet fire and safety standards,

- development of guidelines for the appropriate provision of psychotropic medications,

- development of a policy which would permit involuntary patients to refuse psychotropic medications,

- treatment and placement of mentally retarded mental patients,

- accreditation of the state hospitals by the Joint Commission on Accreditation of Hospitals (JCAH, later changed to Joint Commission on Accreditation of Healthcare Organizations),

- development of specialized programs for the adult general psychiatric patients and geriatric patients,

- development of aftercare plans for patients discharged from the hospitals in a system of community support programs for these patients, and

- the seeking of appropriate funding from the legislature for implementation of these improvements.

An administrative requirement of the Settlement Agreement was the establishment of a three-person review panel to monitor Defendants' compliance with the requirements of the lawsuit. The panel consisted of David Pharis, psychiatric social worker, as the coordinator; James Peden, M.D., psychiatrist; and Martha Boston, attorney, as the two part-time members. In 1988 James Peden, M.D. and Martha Boston left the panel and David Pharis became the Court Monitor.

---

2. R.A.J. v. Miller, Settlement Agreement, April 1981.

The 1981 R.A.J. Settlement Agreement was conceptually a summary of all of the legal issues and standards that had been developed during the previous ten years. It was not as specific as Wyatt v. Stickney, because it did not include staffing ratios, square footage measurement of rooms, and the other prescriptive requirements of that court case, but it did include all of the issues.[3] The agreement therefore was a complex document covering a wide range of clinical and institutional issues.

An evaluation plan, developed as an early organizational task, identified fifty separate requirements. National and local standards and rules were examined which could be used to define compliance. Many areas which did not contain measurement criteria were identified. The Settlement Agreement contained such phrases as: "There will be adequate staff to provide thirty hours of programming per patient to meet their individualized treatment needs" and "clients will receive individualized treatment planning and programming relevant to their treatment needs." The term "substantial compliance" was used throughout the document as a compliance measure. This term, however, was not defined in any way.

In 1981 the Settlement Agreement was considered to be a model of clarity and probably was more clear than some similar documents. However, efforts at implementation and evaluation over the years had painfully indicated that terms such as "individualized treatment" and "substantial compliance" needed operational definitions to enable all participants in the suit to understand what actually constituted compliance.

Implementation of the Settlement Agreement began in 1982 with TXMHMR implementing portions of an action plan and the Review Panel conducting reviews of the hospitals every six months.

The Settlement Agreement required the development of several new policies. One requirement which necessitated innovation was the development of standards for the appropriate use of psychotropic medications. The development of these standards was based upon negotiations conducted primarily between the Defendants' psychiatric consultants and a consultant for the U.S. Department of Justice. Work on these standards began in 1981; in the fall of 1982 a draft policy was presented to the TXMHMR Commissioner for approval.

---

3. Wyatt v. Stickney, 325 F. Supp. 781 (M.D. Ala. 1971).

The Commissioner did not approve the document and expressed his opposition to many of the principles of the policy.

This opposition from the Commissioner caused the negotiation process to break down temporarily. In late fall of 1982 the Review Panel, which up to this point had not been involved in negotiations between the parties, made a formal recommendation to the court that the medication policy developed through the negotiation process should be adopted by the court as the policy which would meet the requirements of the Settlement Agreement. The Defendants strenuously objected to the approval of the policy but began to involve themselves again in the negotiation process, which now included the Review Panel. In February 1983 a Supplemental Agreement regarding the appropriate use of psychotropic medication was filed with the court.[4]

This policy became a TXMHMR rule and has been revised to reflect current medical practice. The policy defined dosage ranges for each major class of psychotropic medication; had specific ranges for adults, children, and geriatric clients; and contained guidelines on how medication usage monitoring should be conducted by the hospitals. The rationale for unusual practices, such as the use of polypharmacy, now required documentation and routine checks for involuntary movements became obligatory.

Another compliance issue required the development of a policy to permit clients to consent to psychotropic medications. The only guideline in the R.A.J. Settlement Agreement was that this policy should be based upon the legal standards of Rennie v. Klein or Rogers v. Okin.[5] The difference between these two cases are explained in Chapter 3. Negotiations took place on this issue during 1983 and 1984. Initially the Plaintiffs and the Review Panel supported a rule based on the due process standards of Rogers v. Okin while Defendants opposed the development of any policy.

In January 1984 the Review Panel filed a recommendation presenting a rule on consent for the administration of psychotropic medications. Both Defendants and Plaintiffs objected to this proposed rule. Plaintiffs maintained that except in the case of an emergency the

---

4. R.A.J. v. Miller, Supplemental Agreement, February 1983.
5. Rogers v. Okin, 634 F. 2d 650 (1st Cir. 1980).
Rennie v. Klein, 720 F. 2d 650 (3rd Cir. 1983).

competent patient had an absolute right to refuse medications. Defendants maintained that the act of involuntary commitment to a state hospital indicated that the patient lacked the judgment necessary to exercise such a right. In essence, Defendants said that committed patients were in fact incompetent to make treatment decisions. Defendants further argued that by restricting the administration of psychotropic medications, which was the primary means of treatment in state hospitals, the rule placed treatment facilities in a position where they were unable to perform their duties.

Further negotiations between the parties and the Panel did not result in an agreed upon policy but rather in the submission of two policies.[6] The Plaintiffs' document supported the absolute right of patients to refuse medications. Modeled after Rogers v. Okin, this policy was supported by the Review Panel. The Defendants submitted a document which used the model of medical review developed through Rennie v. Klein, which permitted the client to request a second medical opinion and to receive such an opinion concerning the medical acceptability of the originally prescribed medication.

In a Memorandum Opinion and Order filed June 22, 1984, Judge Barefoot Sanders ruled that Defendants' proposed rule adequately protected the rights of involuntarily committed patients in light of standards specified in current case law.[7] The TXMHMR policy permitted voluntarily committed patients to refuse medications. If the hospital considered that it could not adequately treat the patient without the use of medications, the hospital could then discharge the patient from care or attempt to obtain an involuntary commitment. Patients in the hospital on an emergency commitment order or an order of protective custody could also refuse medications except in situations of a psychiatric emergency where a physician could force medications.

Patients under two forms of involuntary mental commitment (temporary or extended) could not refuse medications but could object to the medication and receive a second opinion from a hospital psychiatrist other than the patient's treating physician. The second psychiatrist would review the medication, determine the appropriateness of the treatment, and make a determination about whether the patient

---

6. R.A.J. v. Miller, Parties Objections to Review Panel's Recommendation 24, March 1984.

7. R.A.J. v. Miller, Memorandum Opinion and Order, June 1984.

understood the consequences of their decision to refuse the medication. If the physician determined that the patient did understand the consequences, the patient would receive consultation by a third psychiatrist who was an outside consultant. The consultant would make a determination about the psychiatric appropriateness of the treatment. In addition to the provisions reinforcing the professional appropriateness of the treatment, the policy insured that all patients should be educated about the purpose of their medication, its possible side effects, and the nature of alternative methods of treatment.

The Texas policy was complicated and confusing, posing a need for procedural outlines to define proper implementation of the procedures. Mental health advocates who preferred the due process proceedings of Rogers v. Okin rule attacked the rule because it did not recognize an absolute right to refuse medications.

In 1990 Advocacy, Incorporated, the federal protection advocacy agency in Texas, challenged the adequacy of the due process protections of the TXMHMR Consent to Medication Rule. The case was filed in state rather than federal court. The court's findings prompted TXMHMR to negotiate a Settlement Agreement which in turn became state law in 1992. The new law established formal mechanisms for the due process protections of a person's competency. When an involuntarily committed patient objected to medication, the treating physician would make a determination of the person's capacity for informed consent. If the physician determined that the person had the capacity to make the decision, the treatment refusal must be honored and treatment not given. If the physician questioned the patient's capacity for informed consent, the physician could file a petition to the county court for a due process determination of capacity. The court could order medications within large classes—such as antipsychotics, antidepressants, and antianxiety medications—if the court found that the person did not have capacity to make informed consent decisions.

Besides the negotiation of several important rules required by the 1982 Settlement Agreement, the years 1982–1992 represent a time of adversarial conflict between the Parties in the lawsuit and the Review Panel. The Review Panel began its active monitoring in 1982. In December 1983 the Panel submitted its Third Report to the Court concluding that there were four areas of noncompliance with requirements of the Settlement Agreement. These included the lack of individualized treatment, a high degree of aggressive behavior in the hospitals, inadequate staffing, and the fact that mentally retarded patients were not being placed in appropriate facilities.[8] An evidentiary hearing was held in February 1984.

In April 1984 Judge Sanders confirmed the Review Panel's findings of lack of individualized treatment, inadequate staffing, and the high degree of aggressive behavior in the hospitals and determined that the Texas Department of Mental Health and Mental Retardation was out of compliance with requirements of the Settlement Agreement.[9]

Disagreements over the findings from this evidentiary hearing revealed the lack of clarity around the requirements of the Settlement Agreement. After the Court's order of noncompliance there were further agreements aimed at addressing the three areas of noncompliance. Definitions, standards, and performance measures for individualized treatment were developed. Programs dealing with aggressive behavior were implemented at the hospitals. Finally, staffing ratios for mental health workers were put into place at every hospital. Defendants disagreed with the conclusions of the evidentiary hearing and particularly contested the imposition of mandatory staffing ratios.

The 1984 court order mandating staffing ratios necessitated an emergency appropriation of funds from a special session of the Texas Legislature. TXMHMR requested that the Court permit that the staffing ratio requirements could be met by the reduction of patients in the hospitals as well as by hiring staff. The Court accepted this proposal that patients could be discharged to facilities adequately staffed to meet their needs. This court order expanded the Court's jurisdiction over the area of community mental health care.[10]

The development of the "$35.50 per day" program, a mechanism for putting money into the community, became an unanticipated side effect of the staffing requirements. When TXMHMR requested the alternative of complying with staff requirements through the reduction of the population in the hospitals, the Commissioner, Dr. Gary Miller, conceived of a means of transferring the monies which would have been used for the hiring of staff to community programs. The

---

8. R.A.J. v. Miller, Review Panel's Third Report to the Court, December 1983.

9. R.A.J. v. Miller, Memorandum Opinion, April 1984.

10. R.A.J. v. Miller, Order for Stipulated Recommendations of Remedies, June 1984.

specific bed-day population for each mental health authority (MHA) was calculated for a particular baseline period of time. The MHAs then were notified that for each day that they reduced below the baseline utilization rate, they could earn $35.50 per day. The earnings would be calculated on a quarterly basis and payments of funds thereafter were based on the bed-day reduction of the previous quarter.

The $35.50 program created an incentive for MHAs to focus on serving the chronically mentally ill in the community. The emphasis on a reduction of hospital bed days and the need to maintain a reduction were direct results of this program. The $35.50 program provided approximately $38 million of new money into the community mental health system from the summer of 1984 to the summer of 1988.

Public concern was expressed directly to the Court and through the media during the late months of 1984 that TXMHMR was inappropriately dumping clients from the state hospitals to inadequate community resources. One hospital caused adverse publicity by attempting to reduce the length of patients' stay in acute programs through the aggressive use of psychotropic medications. The fact that this hospital actually discharged people and placed them on busses from Austin to Houston with the understanding that they were to go to the local shelter increased the negative public reaction.

An evidentiary hearing to examine the appropriateness of Defendants efforts at reducing the populations of the hospitals was held in March 1985. In June 1985 the Court ruled that there was no evidence of inappropriate discharging of patients on the part of the hospitals.[11] However, the Court concluded that many clients discharged from the hospitals received services which were minimally adequate. The Court found that minimally adequate services did not comply with the court order; the community alternatives must be "adequately staffed facilities sufficient to provide appropriate treatment."[12]

After the court's determination on aftercare, the parties and the Review Panel negotiated definitions of adequate community based aftercare for patients discharged from the state hospitals. Adequate

---

11. R.A.J. v. Miller, Findings of Fact and Conclusions of Law, June 1985.
12. Ibid.

community based aftercare was defined as: appointment with aftercare provider, aftercare plan and effort made to provide the service, follow-up and outreach, case management for all eligible clients, and provision of or referral for nonclinical support services (food, clothing, and shelter).[13] The story of the attempts to determine the adequacy of community aftercare will be told in Chapters 7 and 8.

From 1984 through 1991 the Review Panel and then the Court Monitor submitted an additional eleven monitoring reports to the Court. These reports continued to find problems in the provision of individualized treatment. Defendants usually attempted to deny or discredit the findings of these reports. Over these years progress was recognized in the following areas: achievement and maintenance of JCAHO accreditation, the renovation of the physical plant of the hospitals to meet life safety code requirements, the achievement and maintenance of patient to staff ratio requirements, and the implementation of a clinical peer review process and ongoing staff training procedures. The Monitor recommended that these issues be found in full compliance by the Court and that each issue be discharged from the jurisdiction of the Court.[14]

After the dismissal of four major issues from the jurisdiction of the court the Monitor issued a major compliance monitoring report in 1991 maintaining that problems still existed in the areas of individualized treatment and the protection of patient rights.[15]

Defendants disagreed with many of the findings of the 1991 report. Rather than having an expensive evidentiary hearing to determine the validity of the findings, the parties and the Court Monitor agreed to negotiate means of addressing the core problems that continually caused disagreement over compliance findings. The parties agreed that the main barrier to compliance was lack of specific agreement over what constituted compliance.

These negotiations resulted in the development of a new Settlement Agreement to replace the previous agreement and all court or-

---

13. R.A.J. v. Miller, Recommendation 35, October 1986.

14. R.A.J. v. Miller, Memorandum Opinion and Order on Recommendation 79, January 1991.

15. R.A.J. v. Jones, R.A.J. Review Panel Fourteenth Report to the Court, March 1991.

ders subsequent to it.[16] This agreement was based upon the concept of a self-monitoring system developed by the Texas Department of Mental Health and Mental Retardation called the Continuous Quality Improvement (CQI) System. This system contained instruments to measure each compliance issue, the criteria for the measurement of the issue, and definitions of what constituted compliance for each issue in terms of a numerical compliance score.

The compliance issues to be evaluated included the implementation of the consent to psychoactive medication rule, the provision of individualized treatment and medical treatment, protection of patient rights, compliance with the Department's rule for investigation of abuse and neglect allegations, and the provision of community aftercare requirements. Hospital review teams would monitor these compliance issues each month. The teams would review a ten percent sample of the hospital population. Within a six-month period a sizeable sample would therefore be reviewed which would provide a proportionate picture of the hospital by types of programs. Two state teams composed of community based psychiatrists, other mental health professionals, and mental health advocates would then measure compliance at each hospital once every six months. These teams would do so by reviewing a sample of the cases previously reviewed by the hospital teams. The Court Monitor and his consultants would monitor findings of the state teams and verify these findings.

Compliance would be achieved when a hospital reached the required compliance level on an issue for a six-month period. The issue would then be expected to be maintained in compliance for an additional six-month period of active review by the Court Monitor and then for two six-month periods of continued review by the state's consultants.

This graduated review process aimed at validating the hospital's scores permitted the gradual withdrawal of court supervision once continued compliance had been demonstrated. The process in essence established a series of rewards for establishing and maintaining compliance. It also established a graduated method for Defendants to earn back their autonomous functioning. Through the Quality Systems Oversight (QSO) process, compliance was monitored for four time periods for eight issues at each of the eight state hospitals. Therefore,

---

16. R.A.J. v. Jones, Settlement Agreement, March 1992.

sixty-four separate compliance requirements had to be met for four specific stages of time. Compliance was achieved when a hospital passed the compliance target for a six-month period of active monitoring. Compliance must be repeated for a second six-month period of active monitoring and then continued for a twelve-month period of inactive monitoring at the acceptable compliance level.

The Court approved this new Settlement Agreement as a means of obtaining compliance in this lawsuit in March 1992. Hospital reviews using the new compliance monitoring system began in September of 1992. From September 1992 until October 1997, ten rounds of site visits were made at each of the eight state hospitals. These visits occurred on a six-month revolving schedule. Compliance was established with the first level of requirements in September 1992, when one hospital met the compliance requirements for all eight compliance issues (refer to Charts I, II, III at the end of this chapter). This hospital was also the first hospital to meet the requirements of the second stage of compliance monitoring for seven of its eight issues. It went into the inactive phase of monitoring in April 1993. From then on hospitals established their compliance requirements during the ten consecutive review periods. The first hospital to be discharged from the jurisdiction of the Court, having met all of its compliance requirements, did so in January 1995. The other hospitals had moved toward meeting the requirements, but three hospitals still had not established compliance at the first level of compliance in several areas by January 1995. These areas included individualized treatment, consent to medication, and medication monitoring. In response to the Monitor's expressed concern about these hospitals' lack of capacity to establish compliance in these areas, Central Office of TXMHMR made the innovative suggestion of changing the review schedule to include intensive reviews by a R.A.J. monitor and a QSO monitor on a monthly basis until the hospitals passed the requirements to go into the inactive monitoring phase.

Intensive reviews were done by one consultant from each of the teams on a monthly basis; they read four records, came up with their right-answer agreement about the scores, and explained to the hospital teams the reasons that their score was different than the hospital score. The hospitals responded to the consultation offered in the intensive reviews and the last hospital went into inactive monitoring in April 1997. The final hospital was recognized as meeting all the requirements for dismissal from the jurisdiction of the Court in September 1997 and the Court dismissed R.A.J. v. Gilbert from its jurisdiction on October 14, 1997.

The remainder of the chapter will present analysis of the process of implementation and my ideas about why compliance has been so difficult to achieve. There will also be an examination of the difference between conditions in the hospitals in the early 1980's and today.

By 1992, the Court recognized compliance with requirements of the achievement and maintenance of JCAHO accreditation, the completion of fire and safety code renovations, the improvement in the adequacy of direct care staffing, and the development of clinical peer review and training procedures. In addition, there were the development of standards for the use of psychotropic medications and the development of a policy for consent to medications. Other less tangible issues remained unresolved.

Compliance was first achieved in areas which were concrete. Rules could be written, money could be appropriated for the hiring of staff or the renovation of buildings, and JCAHO standards could be achieved and maintained. JCAHO represents a nationally accepted set of standards in the field of hospital and psychiatric treatment. JCAHO standards, however, periodically change; performance on standards one year does not mean necessarily the same thing that it means another year. The Texas hospitals achieved JCAHO compliance during the late 1970's and maintained that requirement throughout the fifteen-year implementation phase. At the same time hospitals were maintaining JCAHO accreditation, they received very negative reviews by the Monitor's consultants for inadequate clinical care.

It was clear that it was easier to achieve and maintain JCAHO accreditation than it was to achieve compliance with the patient care issues in the lawsuit. Critics of the Panel or Monitor suggested that this was due to the self-serving subjective nature of the monitoring. I maintain, however, that the difference was caused by a more focused look at clinical care. While JCAHO accreditation is based on meeting many administrative and policy requirements that cover all aspects of hospital management, the R.A.J. requirements focused on more specific features of patient care and were often based on professional judgment about the adequacy of specific clinical actions.

JCAHO requirements focus upon the broad components such as program management, patient management, patients' services, and physical plant management. Many requirements can be met by the presence of job descriptions, policies, procedures, and other written documents which explain how the organizational structure is expected to perform. JCAHO accreditation can reflect good organizational management. Many observers of the JCAHO accreditation process believe that over the years the focus has moved away from definitions of psychiatric clinical practice to a medical approach more appropriate to community hospitals. There also has been a focus upon management practices such as the continuous quality improvement processes. JCAHO currently is advocating the development of active continuous quality improvement management systems.

Rules did not exist in the Texas Department of Mental Health system prior to the filing of the lawsuit in 1974. There were no policies about the use of restraint and seclusion, the use of psychotropic medicines, the investigation of abuse and neglect, or any of the other complicated issues that compose day-to-day patient care. As the discovery phase of this case got underway in the 1970s, a first step was the development of patient care rules. By 1982, when the Review Panel began monitoring, there was an elaborate set of such rules establishing standards for patient care. The development of the consent to treatment rule and the development of the rule governing the appropriate use of psychotropic medications added to the set of standards in this area.

There also was progress from 1982 to 1992 in the areas of patient environment and the adequacy of staffing. The contracts to renovate buildings to meet life safety codes greatly changed the patient environment. In 1981 and 1982, the eight Texas state hospitals had populations of approximately 4,200 people at any one time. In 1997 the population was approximately 2,800 patients. In 1982 patients were housed on wards of sixty to ninety patients with a treatment team of one physician, one psychologist, one or two social workers, and some RN's, LVN's, and mental health workers. Many buildings were named units but, because of the architecture of the units, were divided up into six or eight wards which were physically separate from each other. The total number of staff on the unit could sound adequate, but when the number of staff who were serving patients on physically isolated wards was examined, adequacy became another issue. Often one or two people were alone with a group of twenty to forty patients.

The dormitories were large bay areas with twenty to forty beds in a section with no physical partitions. Staff often considered this arrangement positive because they could walk down hallways and see all of the patients in the dorm area. By 1982, this type of arrangement was a violation of a JCAHO standard which required that there be no more than eight people in a room and that there be provisions for privacy.[17]

Patients spent most of their time in large day rooms. There could be sixty to ninety people milling around at any one time. Many people would sit in metal chairs lined up in rigid lines against the wall; others would pace back and forth in either agitated or zombie-like states. The noise level was very high and the air was filled with acrid cigarette smoke. One of the benefits of being a patient in the Texas state hospital system in 1982 was that the state provided cigarettes. Mental patients, therefore, easily became addicted to cigarettes and caffeine, another substance supplied readily in day rooms. The fact that there was little for patients to do in these day rooms other than pace, smoke, and get on each others nerves, contributed to the chaotic antitherapeutic environment that existed at the time.

The Review Panel became concerned about the adequacy of staffing at the hospitals during the spring and summer of 1983 as it investigated employees' complaints about unsafe conditions at several of the facilities. Many of these complaints stated that both clients and employees were placed in unsafe situations because of inadequate staffing.

The 1981 Settlement Agreement required that "patients have the right to have sufficient staff available to provide adequate individualized treatment planning and programming. Staffing shall be in sufficient numbers to adequately care, treat, and habilitate patients so that patients will need to be hospitalized for the shortest possible duration. Specifically, the Defendants shall provide adequate staff support to make available to all patients an average of thirty hours per week of appropriate planned or scheduled activities related to the pa-

---

17. Joint Commission on Accreditation of Hospitals, *Consolidated Standards Manual*, Chicago, IL, 1981, p. 151.

78 State Hospital Reform: Why Was It So Hard to Accomplish?

tient's treatment plan and the unit treatment program." The Settlement Agreement also required that patients be protected from harm which assumes adequate staff to protect patients from themselves and others and to cope with emergencies.[18]

The panel examined what standards defined adequate psychiatric staffing. JCAHO's standards at the time required that the staffing be adequate to meet the needs of client conditions.[19] These standards were not specific in that they did not give ratios or any other criteria for adequacy. I, however, observed an Assistant Deputy Commissioner of Mental Health address the TXMHMR Board about the complaints about inadequate staffing. This official told the TXMHMR Board that the Department's own standards for staffing adequacy were that there should be four mental health workers for every twenty patients on the 7:00 a.m.–3:00 p.m. and 3:00 p.m.–11:00 p.m. shifts, and two mental health workers for every twenty patients on the 11:00 p.m.–7:00 a.m. shift. This translates into a five-to-one patient staff ratio for the day and evening shift and a ten-to-one patient staff ratio for the night shift. These ratios had been developed by TXMHMR's Mental Health Division as standards for budget planning for the annual legislative appropriation request. There were developed for general psychiatric patients and may have been a part of a more comprehensive staffing formula for budget purposes. However, these standards were never implemented by the Mental Health Division because they appeared to be too costly. The standards were presented to the TXMHMR Board as representing a desired staffing ratio. The Review Panel used the five-to-one and ten-to-one ratios as a standard for their report to the court in 1983.[20] In a resulting Third Report evidentiary hearing TXMHMR denied that such standards had ever been adopted by the Department and decried the use of staffing ratios as a means of defining adequacy of staffing.

Armed with the five-to-one and ten-to-one staffing ratios as a guideline, the Review Panel examined staffing at all of the hospitals during the months of July, August, and September 1983. All of the eight state hospitals fell short of five-to-one and ten-to-one staffing

---

18. R.A.J. v. Miller, Settlement Agreement, 1981.

19. Joint Commission on Accreditation of Hospitals, *Consolidated Standards Manual*, Chicago, IL, 1981, p. 18.

20. R.A.J. v. Miller, R.A.J. Review Panel Third Report to the Court, December 1983, p. 29.

guidelines. Analysis of data from the month of August 1983 indicated that hospitals ranged from eight-to-one to twelve-to-one on the first shift, from eight-to-one to fourteen-to-one on the second shift, and from seven-to-one to nineteen-to-one on the third shift.

Since the Review Panel was using the five-to-one and ten-to-one ratio as the definition of minimal requirement for a safe environment, the Panel considered that under no circumstances should a single staff member ever be on a ward alone. Single coverage should be considered dangerous to both patients and staff. A single staff person could not simultaneously deal with the needs of twelve to forty patients. Obviously a lone staff person is unprotected in a violent situation. Routine duties such as checking on secluded or restrained patients every fifteen minutes, dispensing medication, providing one-to-one coverage of suicidal patients, or taking patients on any trips would immediately occupy one staff person per task. This illustrates the inadequacy of even two-person staffing on a unit with very disturbed patients. The units often had as many as six patients on suicidal precautions at one time. If these people required one-to-one observation they were each demanding the use of a staff person. In 1983 when staff coverage was low, wards handled this type of situation by moving suicidal patients' beds into a day room where they could all be observed as a group by a single staff member.

Lone staffing of a ward was not a rare situation in the summer of 1983. In August seventy-seven wards out of one hundred twenty-four, or sixty-two percent, had shifts which were staffed by one person. The Admissions Units of two of the largest hospitals had the highest rate of single person staffing. Two hospitals reported their staffing data in such a way that it was apparent that on the night shifts there was often either no scheduled coverage on a unit or scheduled staff did not report for duty and the end result was lack of coverage for a ward area. One hospital had forty-five different incidents during August 1983 when there was no coverage on a ward. Five were on the 7:00 a.m.–3:00 p.m. shift, twelve were on the 3:00 p.m.–11:00 p.m. shift, and twenty-eight were on the 11:00 p.m.–7:00 a.m. shift. This lack of staffing occurred on fourteen wards with an average census of twenty-two patients. Two wards on an adolescent unit in another hospital had ten incidents where there was no coverage on the 11:00 p.m.–7:00 a.m. shift. In these situations staff had to be pulled from other wards to provide coverage.

The problem of borrowing staff to provide coverage for an understaffed unit was twofold. Borrowing from another ward placed pressure upon the coverage in that ward. Some of these hospitals were so tightly staffed that they could not afford to move staff around. Also when staffing was provided by borrowing, patients were likely cared for by strangers.

The lowest mental health worker coverage occurred on the 11:00 p.m.–7:00 a.m. shift during the week and all three shifts on the weekends. The presentation of the July, August, and September staffing data to the Court convinced Judge Sanders that staffing was inadequate at the state hospitals and prompted him, after an evidentiary hearing in January of 1984, to order that the hospitals meet the five-to-one or ten-to-one staffing ratios.[21] The Department of Mental Health greatly objected to this court order. It disavowed the validity of those specific staffing ratios or any staffing ratios arguing that staffing needs varied depending on conditions of clients.

The Court's determination in April 1984 that there was noncompliance in the areas of lack of individualized treatment, adequacy of staffing, and high degree of aggressive behavior in the state hospitals created a crisis in the Texas Department of Mental Health and Mental Retardation. Defendants did not agree with these findings and they resented the additional requirements that the findings of noncompliance placed upon them. Mandated staffing ratios of five-to-one and ten-to-one placed severe demands on an already tight budget. The Governor was required to call a special session of the legislature and $16.7 million were appropriated on an emergency basis for hiring of an additional 1,095 mental health workers to bring the hospitals up to standards. The Court required that ratios be met by June 15, 1984.[22] TXMHMR requested permission from the court to fill the staffing ratios by either the hiring of staff or by the reduction of patients from the hospitals. The Court granted this request with the stipulation that patients could only be discharged to adequately staffed community facilities. These court orders enlarged the Court's role in community mental health.

During the next several years staffing ratio issues were constantly being negotiated between the Parties and the Panel and compromises

---

21. R.A.J. v. Miller, Memorandum Opinion and Order, April 1984.
22. Ibid, April 1984.

were being submitted to the Court. These compromises ranged from nine specific exceptions to the "two persons per ward" staffing requirement on individual programs with special needs to changing the application of ratios from wards, to units, and ultimately to the entire hospital. From the Defendants' point of view, the broadening of the ratios to the entire hospital permitted some flexibility in staffing. The advantage to this was that a ward with few agitated patients could have less staffing than an acute unit that had constant turnover of very disturbed patients. This conformed to the philosophy supported by JCAHO that staffing should fit the individual characteristics of patients. From the point of view of the Defendants, however, staffing compromises always resulted in reducing costs and reducing the restrictiveness of the regulations. Defendants placed constant pressure upon the Panel and the Plaintiffs' attorneys to make these compromises in the staffing requirements.

The Panel felt somewhat insecure about its basis for staffing requirements. Staffing ratios were not required or supported by JCAHO. These particular ratios were based upon standards developed by TXMHMR which they in turn disowned. These disavowed standards, therefore, seemed a shaky base for this court-ordered requirement. To make matters worse, the Civil Rights Division of the United States Justice Department, after the change from the Carter administration to the Reagan administration, changed its philosophical orientation to these institutional reform lawsuits. After the Romeo v. Youngberg decision in 1982 the Justice Department modified its support on many of the issues in the lawsuit. The Justice Department was particularly nervous about specific staff ratios and began supporting Defendants' requests for modifications of these ratios. Modifications and compromises with the staffing requirement continued from 1985 through January of 1988 when the court approved a proposed statistical method to evaluate TXMHMR's compliance with staff to patient ratios.

This last compromise was constructed by consultants to the Panel after persistent requests from the Defendants for further technical changes. This method examined compliance in terms of average day-to-day performance of each hospital for a six-month period rather than in terms of day-to-day performance. The staffing ratios were altered from the five-to-one and ten-to-one requirement on a ward basis to a four-to-one and eight-to-one on a hospital-wide basis for all hospitals except the geriatric program which was to be staffed at a six-to-one and ten-to-one ratio on a hospital-wide basis. A compromise from the ward basis to a hospital-wide basis was to permit flexibility in staffing from one unit that needed heavier staffing to the unit that could function with lighter staffing. The rationale for moving from the day-to-day compliance requirement to a six-month requirement was that this permitted a degree of flexibility for the manager who was contending with job market fluctuations, illness of staff, and other anticipated but somewhat uncontrollable circumstances. The estimate for the six-month period permitted some fluctuation between good and bad days of staffing. It also permitted the manager to not have to overreact to a day or two of people not reporting to work or to an increase in the census by needing to immediately hire staff.

From January 1988 through January 1991, the hospitals established and maintained compliance with this last version of the staffing-ratio requirements. In January 1991 the court dismissed the staffing-ratio requirements from the lawsuit.[23]

All of the modifications in the staffing-ratio requirements were in the direction of making the requirements less rigorous. The pressure from the Defendants to modify and diminish the restrictiveness of the requirements was persistent and unending until the time that the requirements were recognized as being in compliance and discharged from the jurisdiction of the Court. At that time the Defendants agreed to adhere to the staffing ratios as guidelines. From the Defendants point of view, staffing-ratio requirements obviously represented interference by an outside group upon the management of the hospitals. Defendants always contended that staffing had been adequate and that it was the responsibility of Defendants to determine what safe staffing was.

It is interesting to note that at the same time that the Defendants argued against the need for staffing ratios, they independently developed responsible formulas for determining staffing adequacy in their biannual budget request. This funding formula has been used for budget requests for the last four biannual sessions of the legislature and it gradually has been accepted by the Texas Legislature as an ad-

---

23. R.A.J. v. Miller, Memorandum and Opinion on Recommendation 79, January 1991.

equate funding formula. During the recent legislative sessions, the hospitals were funded by the legislature at approximately 97 percent of the formula. It is important to recognize that the funding formula was done outside the purview of the lawsuit. TXMHMR developed the funding formula as an activity unconnected to the lawsuit compliance but maintained that the funding formula was needed to achieve and maintain JCAHO and R.A.J. lawsuit requirements. The funding formula does establish specific staff ratios for physicians, nurses, psychologists, social workers, activity therapists, and mental health workers.

After the Review Panel established in an evidentiary hearing in 1984 that there was inadequate staffing and a high level of aggressive behavior at the hospitals, TXMHMR was directed to establish means of measuring aggressive behavior at the hospitals on a monthly basis. TXMHMR was very reluctant to do so, probably because it was concerned about the liability and embarrassment that such data might cause. However, an accurate reporting system was created although its potential as a management tool was never fully utilized. It became an information system that was grudgingly developed because of a court order but never appropriately used by hospital management.

During the period aggression data was collected, averages for a six-month period remained fairly consistent over time. The average number of incidents per month was around 3,400 with variations from month to month from 2,800 to 4,200. Out of approximately 3,400 aggressive acts there were 400 to 450 injuries per month. Injuries resulted in 15–20 percent of the reported incidents. Most injuries, however, were not serious and approximately eighty percent to eighty-five percent of these injuries required only minor first aid.[24]

The types of acts committed were very consistent from month to month. Nonsexual assault on staff was always the most frequent type of acts, followed by nonsexual assault on clients, verbal threats, self-assaults, assaults on property, and finally sexual assaults on staff and clients. This appeared to be a very stable pattern over time. The assaults were primarily hitting, biting, and scratching; most did not result in serious injuries and so could be considered nuisance acts. Ap-

---

24. R.A.J. v. Miller, Aggressive Incident Data reported to the Court Monitor from 1985 to 1991.

proximately twenty percent of the patients during any month were responsible for all the aggressive acts.

The analysis of incidents by time of day depicts a bimodal pattern. A high number of aggressive incidents occurred at 8:00 a.m. and again at 5:00 p.m. Very few incidents occurred during sleeping hours and there was also a characteristic mid-day decline in the number of aggressive acts.

Although the overall number of aggressive incidents did not change noticeably over a several year period, there was a reduction in the number of injurious incidents over that period. It is possible that a combination of the reduction in population and the increased numbers of mental health workers available to deal with patients on the ward have made it possible for direct care staff to intervene more quickly and effectively in aggressive acts thus preventing or stopping the acts prior to their becoming serious.

In the fall of 1991, the Defendants petitioned the court to reduce the reporting requirements of aggressive incidents to include only the reporting of injuries caused by aggressive acts. The rationale was the onerousness of the reporting requirements. The Court accepted the request and did reduce the requirement. As of December 1991, aggression reporting requirements only reported serious and nonserious injuries.

The Review Panel's reasons for the request of the monitoring of such aggressive activity, was a belief that these acts did occur frequently, were an integral part of life in the hospitals, and as such presented obligations to the staff to learn about how to manage such behavior. The Panel recognized that most of the time the aggression did not cause injuries. However, at times the nuisance level aggressive behavior which was common in the facilities did provoke much more serious acts of aggression. The most serious examples of this included one murder and a situation where a man gouged out the eyes of another man who had been pestering people with minor but frequent acts of aggression. The Panel's belief that the monitoring of aggressive behavior could be a positive management tool was never accepted by the Defendants and little use was made of these data. This was one of many examples of how the Monitor's concepts of progressive management varied from the beliefs of TXMHMR's administrators. The fact that consultation was offered in the context of the lawsuit often made the consultation unusable.

Improvements in the physical environment were gradual. From 1982 through 1985 construction in old buildings was aimed at dividing the forty- to sixty-bed areas into units that housed four to eight people. Because of fire safety code requirements concerning airflow and air conditioning it was impossible to simply set up floor-to-ceiling walls. Instead partitions, twelve inches above the ground and eighteen to thirty-six inches below the ceiling, were put up. These became privacy partitions and created quasi-rooms. The intent was to have four people in a unit, but during this time period these areas most often accommodated six to eight people. An area contained a bed and a wardrobe that was intended to offer some privacy from the other five to seven people in the area.

These arrangements often challenged the spirit of the JCAHO requirements of bedroom areas that provided privacy for no more than eight people. The partitions stretched some people's definitions of "room" and "privacy."

Gradually all of the wards at all of the hospitals were renovated to this type of arrangement. The one exception to this consisted of two units at the state's geriatric facility which housed bedridden elderly patients. Here the nursing staff liked the large bay area where they could walk up and down corridors and see the people they were taking care of. The nurses strenuously resisted the partitions into smaller living spaces. This resistance went on for about eight years until the hospital sought financing from the legislature to build a modern facility with semiprivate rooms.

The improvements in the environment have continued to the present time and many wards at each of the hospitals have been remodeled to include semi-private rooms and even single rooms. Most of the partitioned walls are gone and true wall have been constructed. It is unusual at this point to find patients sleeping more than four to a room. The patients' furniture still only includes a bed and a wardrobe, but many patients display pictures and personal belongings.

The environment in dayrooms also improved over the years. In buildings where the same large dayrooms are still in use, these rooms often have been divided by furniture or partitions into smaller living spaces. Other dayrooms have been remodeled into much smaller areas that are equivalent to family rooms in a house. Furnishings are less institutional and more homelike. All of the hospitals have turned the buildings into nonsmoking areas. Patients now go out into enclosed outside areas for fifteen-minute smoking breaks. Smoking remains a very routinized part of hospital life. Smoking privileges are often used as rewards or punishments in that people often lose smoking privileges for minor infractions of rules. There is no question, however, that the air in the buildings has improved tremendously and that the quality of life related to the quality of air has improved.

At the time of the filing of the lawsuit in 1974 many of the most egregious examples of poor care were the misuse and overuse of psychotropic medications. In 1980 when the United States Department of Justice filed expert reports about conditions in the hospitals, there were again many examples of poor use of psychotropic medications. These included overdoses, misuses of medication, and polypharmacy.

Polypharmacy is the use of more than one medication in the same chemical class. If Thorazine is considered to be helpful for schizophrenia, then hypothetically doses of Thorazine, Stellazine, and Haldol could be doubly or triply effective. The error in this idea is that with more than one medication the effectiveness of a single drug is masked. It is difficult to identify either the benefits or the negative side effects that can be attributable to each individual medications. Although polypharmacy was not prohibited in the 1960s and 1970s it is currently considered a poor practice. Current standards caution against it unless there is some specific reason documented in the physician's order.

Prior to 1974 there were no accepted standards for the use of psychoactive medication other than the *Physician's Desk References* or the guidelines given by pharmaceutical companies. The Department of Mental Health did not have standards for the use of psychoactive medications.

As has been discussed earlier in this chapter, the development of such standards was a controversial first step in the implementation of some of the major requirements of this suit. These guidelines included protections against the side effects of the medications. For example, tardive dyskinesia—involuntary movements of the mouth, tongue, arms, and legs caused by neuroleptic medication—can become severe and irreversible. The guidelines require the periodic screening for such movements with resulting reductions in the dosages once movements are identified.

Once the standards for the use of psychoactive medications and the rules for consent to medication were put into practice, the use of medications in the state hospitals became rational and well within the limits of the standards. Physicians are not prohibited from using dosages which are beyond the upper limits for each medication nor are they prohibited from doing polypharmacy, but in each case they must justify the rational for the practice. Their actions are subject to supervisory and peer review. The setting of standards and the subsequent professional scrutiny has reduced the use of high dosages and almost extinguished the incident of polypharmacy. Polypharmacy rarely occurs these days and when it does there is almost always a justifiable clinical rational for its use. Clients are screened for involuntary movements. For a while the R.A.J. consultants questioned the validity of such screening but increased training in the use of screening techniques seemed to have improved the quality of this endeavor.

Progress in the area of providing humane and adequate non-medically-oriented psychiatric treatment has been much more slowly achieved. The R.A.J. Review Panel began questioning the value of individualized treatment in their First and Second Report to the Court. By the Third Report to the Court, eighteen months after the beginning of monitoring, the Panel took a strong position that treatment was not individualized in the state hospitals.[25] Hospital reviews conducted from April through November 1982 indicated that active programming was far less evident on general psychiatric units than on units such as multiple disability programs for mentally retarded/mentally ill clients, or the children and adolescent unit.

In the general psychiatric units patients were often found unoccupied in day rooms. On several units patients were sleeping on the floor because the dorms were locked during the day. With some frequency, direct care staff appeared to be occupied in nursing stations, rather than interacting with the patients. Programming that was taking place on general psychiatric units most often was group activities which permitted little individualized interaction between patient and staff and afforded patients little opportunity for therapy or learning.

---

25. R.A.J. v. Miller, Aggressive Incident Data reported to the Court Monitor from 1985 to 1991.

88 State Hospital Reform: Why Was It So Hard to Accomplish?

Examples of this were group sings, group trips to town, bus trips aimed at taking patients around the community, bingo games in the dayroom, and large classes which involved patients in low-level skill activities, often using children's art materials which were inappropriate for the adult's age level. Individualization of programming was usually not evident. Everybody seemed to be engaged in the same activities at the same times. Treatment plans often had routinized similarity to them with no explanations of how the prescribed activity would be therapeutic to the individual patient. Some programs had daily schedules for all patients with activities such as wake up, grooming, and hand checks to determine whether patients had washed their hands.[26]

One of the original requirements of the R.A.J. Settlement Agreement was the provision of thirty hours of programming per week relevant to patients' needs. This provision was an attempt to deal with the mindless boredom that was often a part of custodial institutional life. There was a belief that these activities should be therapeutic and aimed at the development of living skills needed for improved functioning. The provision of activities that are truly useful to patients remained a challenge for each hospital. The common approach was to set up classes that patients could attend. To some extent these resembled classes on a community college campus, which may well be an appropriate model for such activity. Patients who were restricted to their units had classes on the unit. Patients who had grounds privileges attended classes in centralized rehabilitation programs. These were usually in nice facilities with gyms, a swimming pool, woodworking, arts and crafts, and a number of rooms that contain kitchens, apartments, stores, and other environments that model normal life. The intent of these classes was to help the patient learn to function in the community or to function better in their hospital environment.

Classes ranged from medication management, symptom management, reality orientation, individual therapy, group therapy, ward government, arts and crafts, music appreciation, sex education, substance abuse groups, sexual abuse groups, and activities which are called adult living skills. These could include grooming, money management, and learning the bus system in the community. There were

---

26. R.A.J. v. Miller, Aggressive Incident Data reported to the Court Monitor from 1985 to 1991.

The History of the R.A.J. Lawsuit in Texas 89

always a large number of recreational activities that were generally called leisure time activities. Over the years hospital staff resisted accepting the need for thirty hours of programming. The resistance remained so adamant that in the negotiation of the new 1992 Settlement Agreement the requirement was reduced to twenty hours of programming relevant to the individual's treatment needs. This issue of providing psychosocial rehabilitation will be discussed in more detail in Chapter 10.

Why was it difficult for the hospitals to do individualized treatment and to develop meaningful treatments or programs for the psychiatric patients? Reasons for this could be the subjective nature of the theories about the causes of mental illness and the techniques of psychiatric treatment. There are many competing theories which include psychodynamic, behavioral, learning, psychobiological, and psychosocial explanations of the causes of mental illness and rationales for curative approaches. Some of these theories are backed by empirical research. Others are backed by theory and practitioners often accept one line of research or theory but not another. Stigmas about mental illness abound. These include judgments that people are malingering, that they don't have a will to get better, and that they are sick because there is some internal flaw in their personality or character. Even some of the more scientifically based information about the biological components of mental illnesses can suggest that there is not much hope for improvement and that the most that can be expected is stabilization on medication and maintenance of people in fairly comfortable environments.

The lack of clarity about what can be expected from the treatment of mental illness may be as good an explanation as any for the fact that it took up to fifteen years for the Parties in this court case to make any positive changes in psychiatric practices in the hospitals. Lack of definition of adequate treatment and the constitutional guideline added by the Youngberg v. Romeo court decision which suggested that any professional judgment of a physician is adequate set the stage for rabid adversarial disagreements over what should be considered adequate psychiatric treatment.

The administration of the Texas Department of Mental Health and Mental Retardation system often resented being in the position of having the Federal Court and its monitor exerting any influence or control over its operations. The Monitor's consultants' attempts to consult on clinical or management issues often were not accepted by TXMHMR staff due to the pervasive toxic, adversarial atmosphere of the suit.

One Commissioner, Dr. Gary Miller, clearly did not agree with the Plaintiffs or the Court that conditions existed in 1981 which warranted the requirements of the Settlement Agreement and subsequent Court interventions. He disagreed openly with the findings of the Review Panel. He eloquently presents his position concerning the negative effects of this litigation in Chapter 5. The second Commissioner, Dennis Jones, agreed with some of the objectives of the suit, considered that existing funding was inadequate to meet service needs, and sought increased funding. The third Commissioner, Don Gilbert, conceptually developed the Continuous Quality Improvement process which has proved to be the mechanism which has brought compliance to previously unresolved issues. He describes the positive and negative effects of operating within the confines of the lawsuit in Chapter 6.

While comparing conditions in the hospitals in the 1980s to conditions present in the 1990s, I believe that there has been an ongoing evolution of operational definitions of compliance with the various requirements of this lawsuit which eventually led to the achievement of the objectives of this suit. The following analysis will address questions of why it has taken fifteen years to make major progress towards compliance implementation and why progress has occurred now when it previously had not. The question of why the Defendants turned towards quality improvement concepts as the mechanism for achieving progress in this lawsuit will also be addressed.

Antipsychiatry beliefs did not motivate the actions and policies within the R.A.J. institutional reform litigation. The Parties in this case always accepted that mental illness exists and that there are technologies within the profession of psychiatry aimed at properly managing and treating these illnesses. The disputed question of this lawsuit was not whether mental illness existed but whether adequate care was being provided patients in the state hospitals. At times there was strenuous disagreement over this question. The Plaintiffs always maintained that services were inadequate. Most often the Defendants maintained that services were adequate. However, once the 1981 Settlement Agreement was written, there was publicly expressed consensus by the various actors that the focus of the lawsuit was to improve services.

The History of the R.A.J. Lawsuit in Texas   91

This Settlement Agreement therefore was based upon the premise that the Parties would operate in good faith toward the achievement of mutually desired goals. During the first three years of the lawsuit there was much shared rhetoric between the Parties and the Review Panel that everybody had the same goals and was working in the same direction. After the Review Panel made allegations of noncompliance in four substantive areas and the Court found noncompliance in three areas, this spirit of cooperation was dampened considerably. However, as the Parties became involved in the creation of corrective action plans, some belief in the shared good faith of the Parties returned. From 1984 until 1992 there was always some tension caused by attitudes of trust versus distrust between the attorneys. Nevertheless, the acceptance that people were working together in good faith to obtain compliance remained an integrating concept that encouraged continued work and continued negotiations.

The process of attempting to effect change through a class action lawsuit establishes structural processes which are unique to the legal system. The fact that a court case is settled implies that there will not be a finding of guilt and that there will be agreed-upon plans for remedies which should be acceptable to all parties. The objective of a settlement therefore is not an establishment of a win or lose position but rather the establishment of a win-win process. The existence of a long-term implementation process with a monitoring mechanism establishes the longitudinal process where there will be monitoring, presentation of findings, negotiations about the findings, the development of corrective actions, and continued monitoring. This cycle is expected to lead toward the resolution of the case. This entire process has to go on within the context of good faith or it will become nonfunctional. The parties in this process all have specified roles. The attorneys are to represent the best interest of their clients. The Court Monitor has to objectively monitor the implementation of the compliance requirements and also advocate for the proper implementation of these requirements. The Judge moves the process along and makes determinations about actions that have obstructed the process and finally about whether the process has been successful.

This focus upon negotiation within a context of good faith does not negate the fact that the process is extremely adversarial. The fact that the parties are to represent the best interests of their clients establishes this adversarial position. The situation is exacerbated by the fact that the sanctions from the Court toward the Defendants can be severe. The presentation of critical monitoring was always met with attempts by TXMHMR to discredit and minimize the findings. Negotiations over policies were always strenuously argued.

The atmosphere within the R.A.J. litigation from 1981 until 1990 was a strange combination of overtly expressed good faith and adversarial actions. The process of monitoring, negotiation, corrective action, and further monitoring was also characterized by monitoring, disagreement over findings, and attempts to discredit the impact of findings or change the direction of the case through the negotiation process. It was clear for several years that a Commissioner, his Board, and the attorneys for the Defendants did not agree with many of the requirements of the case or with the monitoring findings.

The change in leadership at TXMHMR did reduce this adversarial position. The adversarial atmosphere was reduced further after the implementation of the 1992 Settlement Agreement, apparently because of improved relationships between the attorneys, increased belief in the good faith efforts of all of the parties involved, and the demonstration by the Defendants of the assumption of responsibility for the achievement of the compliance through the implementations of the quality improvement process.

The reason behind the adoption of the Continuous Quality Improvement System as the mechanism for implementing compliance requirements and compliance monitoring by TXMHMR was the belief that CQI is a state-of-the-art management system which encourages the systemic understanding of the processes by which a service is provided. The CQI system encourages that the people who do the work will actively participate in determining how their work can be done to insure the highest-quality product. There is a delegation of responsibility and authority to each level within the system. Analysis of the processes is based upon objective data. The monitoring system developed by the Defendants therefore is organized to develop an adequate understanding of work processes; to produce accurate, timely, consistent data concerning performance in major compliance areas; and to produce analysis of levels of performance with specific expectations for improvement.[27]

---

27. Texas Department of Mental Health and Mental Retardation Quality System Oversight Plan, February 1992.

From the perspective of the Court Monitor, interested in obtaining compliance with the requirements of the lawsuit, the Department's focus upon quality improvement as the means of achieving compliance was important primarily in that the Department had developed strategies and management mechanisms for compliance. The acceptance of such a management mechanism represented the assumption of responsibility for the attainment of compliance. This assumption of responsibility was more definitive than any previous effort at compliance.

The implementation of the QSO system did resolve the court case but not without much continued negotiations and the resolution of many barriers to implementation. During an intense seven-to-nine-month negotiation process which produced the QSO system and the eight measurement instruments, the chief negotiator for TXMHMR would occasionally pass the Court Monitor handwritten notes which contained rude salutations. This type of horseplay surprisingly lessened the tension between the two, and the attorneys and the professionals were able to negotiate the QSO Settlement Agreement. The following two years of implementation was a period in which the consultants for TXMHMR and the consultants for the Court Monitor had to resolve strong feelings of distrust. The consultants for the Monitor were convinced that the state would reduce the vigor and validity of standards and would push for early compliance in a manner that was not meaningful. Consultants for TXMHMR were just as convinced that the Monitor and his consultants would do everything to drag out the lawsuit.

During the design phase for the QSO process the attorneys and the Monitor agreed that Doug Hancock, the R.A.J./QSO Coordinator, and I would interview all of the consultants being considered for the QSO teams and that we would jointly agree to the membership of both of the teams. Many of the R.A.J. consultants had been working for me for a number of years. These people were accepted although the Defendants certainly reserved the right to object about any consultant's participation. All new consultants, whether they ultimately went to the QSO teams or to the Monitor's team, were jointly screened and accepted by both of us. Membership in the teams included psychiatrists, psychologists, social workers, psychiatric nurses, physician internists, and client advocates who often were either mental health consumers who had become client advocates or family members representing the Texas Alliance for the Mentally Ill. We initially conducted several training sessions where reviewers were told about the instruments and the criteria for scoring the instruments through presentations on the various rules that the instruments were based upon. The reviewers then scored instruments, determined right answers, and compared their scores with each other. This set up an immediately strained atmosphere because the instruments had been developed through tense negotiations between attorneys and mental health practitioners and from these authors' perspectives the instruments were set in stone.

Now, however, the users of the instruments were expressing initial anxiety and concerns about them. Some clarifications were immediately worked out but for the most part the reviewers were asked to live with the instruments, go through the pilot test at two hospitals, and then begin the reviews in September 1992. The reviewers' anxiety about their new roles and about the criteria for making judgments about the instruments continued through the pilot tests of two hospitals and probably through the first round of site visits. During the pilot visits there was open conflict between some of the R.A.J. reviewers and the QSO reviewers. R.A.J. reviewers were seen as hardliners and as somewhat of an elite crew that obviously already had an esprit de corps. Again there was the distrust between the two groups about motivations and intentions. The Director of the R.A.J./QSO Office, Doug Hancock, was faced with the task of setting up two teams of hospital reviewers, training them, giving them a sense of confidence and identity, and at the same time making them acceptable to the hospitals where they would do external reviews. He hoped that the QSO reviewers could be seen not in the negative, authoritative manner that the Monitor's reviewers had been viewed in the past; but of course these reviewers were doing the same job, were working with the Court Monitor's team, and did have to present the findings of the reviews. TXMHMR incorporated the language of total quality improvement and Mr. Hancock was the disseminator of much of this language. Problems were no longer called problems but "opportunities for improvement." R.A.J. consultants, who had experienced their problem identifications being ignored in the past, were skeptical that the word changes would create much of a different environment. They also were somewhat suspicious that the word changes covered an intent to diminish the seriousness of the reviewers' messages to the hospitals.

The pilot tests and the first round of site visits were a time of intense discomfort. It was also a time when the two teams began to develop relationships with each other and began to work out the definitions of compliance and establish more consistent criteria necessary for consistent case reading.

By the end of the second round of site visits the QSO teams had developed a sense of identity and both groups had worked out many of the questions of how to score issues. Unfortunately, one of the mechanisms for resolving these questions of specific scoring problems was ad hoc decision making on the part of Doug Hancock and me during site visits. Consultants would identify some unique situation, not be sure how to score it, and come to us for decisions. We attempted to identify scoring principles and to write down the principle and the scoring decision so that it could be disseminated for the next round. We were not always successful with this. Many of these issues came up time and time again and eventually there were resolutions that were clarified through written material and disseminated to the hospitals. But, there also were experiences where inconsistencies occurred. In the early days there were certainly scores that were inconsistent from one hospital to the other and there was frustration on the part of consultants who were clearly trying to work out conscientious understanding of their jobs. Over time these inconsistencies were resolved through written memos, training conferences, and other communication processes.

The patient rights advocates were the group who may have experienced the most confusion and frustration over the development of consistent criteria for scoring their instruments. It was probably due to the fact that although all of the reviewers had considered themselves patient advocates, many of them had had little experience with the Department's rules. They had to deal with their own reactions to what they were seeing or reading about in the hospitals and they had to continually question what they were seeing in the light of complicated rules. Hours were spent discussing the differences between rights restrictions and rights violations. Texas patient rights rules permitted the restrictions of many behaviors that were otherwise protected by these rules if there was a clinical justification by the treating physician. Such a clinical rationale would create a rights restriction. The absence of such a clinically based rationale would turn the situation into a violation. This was a difference that had to be talked through by both of the reviewers and then the reviewers had to explain this carefully to hospital staff before there were noticeable changes in the treatment of patients on the wards.

The hours of discussion that went on between the two review teams over the series of site visits ultimately resolved many of the disagreements over criteria and the sense of distrust over adversarial positions and developed a relatively consistent approach to reviewing these issues in the hospitals. The two teams also developed trust in the integrity of the system and the motivation of the individual team members. Eventually, the teams functioned as groups of professionals reflecting consistent standards by which they were measuring the state hospitals. As the teams developed confidence in their own measurement and became more consistent in interpreting these criteria to the hospital review teams, the scores between the hospitals and the QSO and R.A.J. reviewers became closer and closer. At this point there is often remarkable consistency between the way the hospitals review themselves and the way that the QSO reviewers score them.

This success in developing consistent, reliable reviewing is one of the strengths of the QSO process. It demonstrates the integrity of some of the design principles of the process. Specifically, the idea that TXMHMR intended to take responsibility for meeting the unresolved requirements of the lawsuit through the development of such a measurement system has been proven. The fact that review teams can come together, read records, and develop consensus understanding of quality of care has also been demonstrated.

Judge David Bazelon in his decision in Rouse v. Cameron discusses the difficulties inherent in a federal court becoming involved in ordering technical reforms in the area of psychiatry. He writes: "Courts are not as competent as hospitals to make treatment decisions. The evaluation of standards of adequacy and suitability may be next to impossible in the present state of psychiatry where 'treatment' means different things to different psychiatrists. No matter how much compulsive treatment is afforded, compulsory hospitalization is itself generally based on ill conceded standards and goals and ought to be reformed radically or discontinued all together. The real problem is one of inadequate resources, which the courts are helpless to remedy—the question posed is one for the legislature and is a basic policy judgment involving overall priorities in the allocation of scarce resources."[28]

Judge Bazelon's point about the inappropriateness of involuntary commitment was not addressed by this lawsuit. At this point the implementation of the R.A.J. litigation appears to have adequately addressed three of Judge Bazelon's concerns. The federal court never assumed the role of substantive decision maker for psychiatry. Implementation of the R.A.J. Settlement Agreement remained in the hands of the Defendants. Monitoring was done by experts in the field of psychiatry and the Court Monitor made recommendations aimed at advancing the implementation of the goals of the case. Decision making and responsibility for implementation, however, always firmly remained in the hands of the Defendants.

The findings of the Court Monitor's expert consultants were often attacked by the Defendants. Debates over professional judgment did occur and often were stumbling blocks in the resolution of issues. However, the development of the QSO process created a system where experts worked together using similar criteria and came to remarkably similar conclusions. The success of this review process suggests that comparably trained professionals using community standards can come up with very congruent conclusions about quality. The success of this process may contribute new meaning to the Romeo v. Youngberg standard that treatment is to be provided within a range of acceptable professional judgment.[29] The fact is that mental health professionals can repeatedly review cases and have similar conclusions about the quality of care.

Judge Bazelon's point that the lack of financial resources is the responsibility of state legislators has also finally been addressed through this court case. The Monitor had repeatedly advocated for the adequate funding of the court case and during recent legislative sessions the legislature responded to the Defendants' request for funds. At this time the hospitals are funded at a level that should support compliance and the question of compliance is no longer based upon the existence of adequate funds. It now should be primarily a question of adequate management and competent performance.

---

28. Bazelon, D., in D. Burris (ed.), *The Right to Treatment* (New York, 1969).
29. Youngberg v. Romeo, 457 U.S. 307 (1982).

Problems of compliance with lawsuit requirements over the years seem to have been caused primarily by disagreements over compliance findings and by disagreements over the meaning of compliance requirements and the criteria for recognizing compliance. Resolution of many of these problems has been achieved through the negotiation of precise definitions of compliance and the measures for establishing compliance. The establishment of community based review teams that look for the rationale for treatment appears to produce consensus about treatment performance.

Chapter 5

Reform through Litigation:
A Commissioner's Perspective

Gary E. Miller

Upon my appointment as Commissioner of the Texas Department of Mental Health and Mental Retardation in February 1982, the R.A.J. class action lawsuit sprang to life. Originally filed in 1974, R.A.J. had remained dormant for several years, discovery continuing until 1980. A Settlement Agreement was negotiated by the parties and approved by U.S. District Judge Barefoot Sanders in 1981. Shortly after my arrival in Texas, Judge Sanders authorized a three-person R.A.J. Review Panel to monitor implementation of the Settlement Agreement, inaugurating a period of change and controversy in the Department. Dramatic improvements took place in the state mental health system, but the improvements were accompanied by vigorous disputes between the Review Panel, Plaintiff's attorneys, and the Department. The strife and controversy persisted throughout the six years of my tenure as Commissioner and for several years after my resignation in 1988.

The R.A.J. lawsuit, then styled R.A.J. v. Miller, and a class action lawsuit filed in the same year and seeking improvements in mental retardation services (Lelsz) dominated my commissionership, occupying huge amounts of my time and energy, and resulting in much personal frustration. My attitude toward and reaction to R.A.J. can best be understood in light of my experience as a public administrator prior to my appointment.

For fifteen years I had held executive positions in mental health agencies in several states, acquiring a reputation as a reformer of public mental health systems and a strong advocate for patient rights. As Deputy Commissioner for Mental Health Services in Texas (1967-1970), my staff and I supervised a major restructuring of state hospitals, established the first community mental health centers in Texas, and initiated the earliest formal linkages between state hospitals and community programs.[1, 2, 3] As Assistant Commissioner of Mental Hygiene in New York state responsible for the western New York region (1970-1972), my staff and I negotiated a then unusual integrated consortium of institutional and community based services for people with mental illness and mental retardation.[4] While still employed by New York state I was telephoned by then Governor Jimmy Carter of Georgia who told me he wished to bring reform to the Georgia mental health system and offered me the job of State Mental Health-Mental Retardation Director.

During my tenure as Commissioner in Georgia, we established the first internal rights protection program for patients in a state mental health system, the Personal Advocacy Unit.[5, 6] This program became the model for others established throughout the country. My staff and I completely restructured Georgia's mental health system so that people with serious mental illnesses could receive treatment in their local area rather than being shipped to Central State Hospital in Milledgeville, which had been the previous practice.[7, 8, 9] The average daily census of Central State Hospital when I came to Georgia was 7,200; that number dropped to under 4,000 in less than two years as a result of the statewide restructuring. This reform was vitally necessary but politically risky as was our campaign to end the horrendous conditions and inhumane treatment suffered by residents of Central State Hospital. My staff and I endured repeated personal and political attacks for extending a modicum of freedom to Central State Hospital patients and demanding that they be provided with such essentials as towels, clean linens, toilet paper and toilet seats.[10, 11, 12] As Director of Mental Health and Mental Retardation Services for New Hampshire for five years prior to my returning to Texas, my staff and I were successful in implementing a statewide patient rights protection system, a statewide case management system, and a shift of services and resources from the state hospital to the community.[13, 14]

I knew about R.A.J. when I accepted the position of Commissioner in Texas, but naively assumed that those who had brought the lawsuit and I would be allies. I believed that we could work together to achieve the goals of the agency and the lawsuit which I considered to be the same—improving treatment and conditions in the state hospitals, assuring patient rights, and shifting resources and patient care from the state hospitals to the community.

During my tenure, I gradually became disillusioned, acquiring an attitude toward R.A.J. which was less than positive. The experience was especially painful to me because any reservations I expressed about the methods or conclusions of the Review Panel or the Court led to my being characterized as one who opposed improvements in mental health treatment and who espoused maintenance of the status quo. Since I struggled throughout my career to improve the lives of people with mental disabilities, I was angered by the unfair and inaccurate claims that I was opposed to progress and that I was dragging my feet in implementing needed reforms.

As Texas' Mental Health and Mental Retardation Commissioner, I worked hard to restructure and rationalize the delivery system, improve treatment of patients, and enhance the human rights of everyone in the agency's care. Substantial improvements were made in all of these areas. The R.A.J. lawsuit may have contributed indirectly to some of the improvements, but most were the result of the commitment, hard work and creativity of the excellent staff of the state agency.

Despite disagreements, we made every effort to work cooperatively with the Review Panel and Plaintiffs in R.A.J. My staff and I bent over backward to comply with all of the requirements imposed by the lawsuit. Our problem was that compliance was a moving target. The Panel, with the Court's blessing, repeatedly interpreted provisions of the Settlement Agreement in new ways, making it difficult for the state agency to know what was expected of it. At no time did I or anyone on my staff suggest that we should disregard or defy any provision of the Settlement Agreement or any Court Order. I appeared frequently before the legislative committees and other bodies to request funds necessary to carry out lawsuit requirements.

During the first two years of my tenure as Commissioner, compliance with R.A.J. seemed to be a reachable goal, despite the amorphous and constantly changing nature of the demands being placed on the Department. A Court Order of March 30, 1984[15] ended what remained of my optimism. I recall my sense of shock and disbelief upon reading the Court Order. I could not fathom how an ostensibly fair and impartial Court could have stretched the plain meaning of the words in the Settlement Agreement to endorse unfounded claims of the Review Panel and fashion arbitrary remedies out of whole cloth. The March 30, 1984 Order was pivotal in changing the course of R.A.J. and the state agency. I shall discuss the order and the events that led to it.

The Review Panel filed with the Court on December 1, 1983, a report highly critical of the Department's state hospitals. The Department acknowledged its shortcomings in several areas but presented strong testimony at a February 3, 1984 hearing that some key conclusions of the Panel were without foundation. The Panel reported that based on its review of patient records, it "had become increasingly concerned about the effectiveness of the treatment which patients are receiving." The thrust of the Panel's complaint was that treatment was not sufficiently "individualized." Scheduled programs and therapeutic activities were typically provided to groups of patients despite the alleged differences in their problems that, according to the Panel, should have resulted in individualized treatment activities.

The state's expert witness, Tracy Gordy, M.D., of Austin and I testified that psychosocial programming affords benefits to patients with a broad range of problems and, by its very nature, focuses on specific problems of patients that are brought forward in group settings. We also emphasized the importance of modern pharmacotherapy in treatment of mental illness, an aspect of treatment addressed only negatively and in a proscriptive fashion by the Panel.

Dr. Gordy and I noted that language used by hospital staff members in the Department's Problem Oriented Record System (PORS) could be improved and refined. Nevertheless, we emphasized that the problem identification and prescribed interventions used in the Department's PORS were consistent with contemporary standards of medical record keeping. The Joint Commission on Accreditation of Hospitals (since renamed the Joint Commission on Accreditation of Healthcare Organizations) agreed with us. Having reviewed medical records from the same facilities, the Joint Commission consistently determined that all of Texas' state hospitals met the Commission's standards with respect to medical record keeping and all other areas. Nevertheless, the Court concurred with the Panel's conclusion that the Department's record keeping was deficient and that we were out of compliance with the Settlement Agreement.

A second area of concern discussed by the Panel in its December 1, 1983 report was an excess of alleged "violence" in the state hospitals. The Panel averred that aggressive acts by severely mentally ill patients could be predicted and prevented by an understanding of "the dynamics and meaning of behavior." Aside from its naive pop psychological analysis, the Review Panel provided no substantiation for its claim, merely putting forward its opinion that excessive violence was occurring.

The Department had for many years employed strategies to reduce injuries and violence in its facilities. The Prevention and Management of Aggressive Behavior (PMAB) Program, was adopted by private psychiatric hospitals in Texas and by the mental health departments of several other states and countries. All direct care employees of the Department were trained in PMAB techniques.

The Department had prepared for several years injury reports documenting the number, type, and severity of injuries in all Department facilities. These routine injury reports were the only conceivable sources of data for the Panel's conclusion about excessive violence. Contrary to the Panel's claim, the reports demonstrated a progressive decline in the rate of serious injuries. Moreover, the vast majority of the injuries reflected in the statistics were not the result of aggressive acts, but of minor accidents.

To overcome the lack of substantiation for its claim of excessive violence, the Panel emphasized in its report a tragic incident that had occurred several months earlier. A previously docile state hospital patient gouged out the eyes of another patient, an aggressive individual who was being held in restraints. The Panel did not discuss the circumstances surrounding this incident or the factors that might have led to it, but instead used it as emotional leverage for its position, implying that it was but one of many violent acts occurring in the state hospitals. As in the case of other reports critical of the Department, the Panel distributed its report to the press and gave media interviews. Panel members emphasized their claim of excessive violence, repeatedly citing the incident of the patient whose eyes were gouged out.

The Panel and the Court faced another problem. There was no language in the Settlement Agreement upon which a claim of excessive violence could reasonably be based. The Court overcame this problem, repeating in its order the account of the patient whose eyes were gouged out and finding the state agency "guilty" of excessive violence as charged by the Panel. The sections of the Settlement Agreement upon which the Court ostensibly based its conclusions bore little if any relationship to the charge of excessive violence.

The first section cited by the Court was the one requiring individualized treatment programming and the availability of 30 hours per week of program activities. It was the clause upon which the finding of inadequate individualized treatment planning, discussed above, was based.

The second section, one requiring a "clean and safe environment," was specifically intended by the parties in the lawsuit to refer to physical surroundings. The Panel and Court maintained that it encompassed violent acts; however, the words of the Settlement Agreement belie that claim. I quote Section 16 in its entirety so that the words speak for themselves:

> 16. Patients shall be entitled to reside in facilities which are environmentally clean and safe. Pursuant to an established routine maintenance and repair program, the physical plant at each facility shall be kept in a continuous state of good repair and operation in accordance with the needs of the health, comfort, safety and well being of the patients.

The Court, determined to support its Review Panel, accepted the Panel's unfounded claim of excessive violence in the hospitals, basing its conclusion on a creative reinterpretation of the language of the Settlement Agreement.

The third deficiency reported by the Panel was insufficient staffing of the state hospitals. My staff and I were in agreement that staffing at all levels needed to improve. I had argued vigorously for additional positions before the Legislative Budget Board and several committees of the 1983 Texas Legislature and would do so again during the July 1994 special session of the legislature.

The Court also found the Department in noncompliance with provisions of the Settlement Agreement requiring adequate staffing levels as it had in the matter of individualized treatment planning and excessive violence. In the case of staffing, the Court went further, imposing a rigid staffing formula for mental health workers (psychiatric aides). The Department was required to meet mental health worker to patient ratios of 1:5, 1:5, and 1:10 on the three shifts on every ward of every state hospital. No evidence was presented at the February 3, 1984 hearing to support these or any other staff to patient ratios. The Panel contended that the ratios were obtained from Department standards, but the Department had neither developed nor proposed staffing ratios for its facilities. Since no source for the ratios could be identified at the February 3, 1984 hearing, the Court Order claimed that the ratios were based on the "professional judgment" of the Panel.

Because of the multiple variables that determined needed staffing levels, the Department, like the joint Commission on Accreditation of Hospitals, had abandoned fixed staffing ratios. Institutional superintendents had based their staffing requirements on multiple factors such as patient numbers, type and acuity; programming requirements imposed by the Department and the R.A.J. Settlement Agreement; and the number and physical layout of the various wards and units. As a result of the Court's venture into micromanagement of the state mental health system, directors of nursing and nursing supervisors in the state hospitals lost their ability to modify staffing levels based on changing needs and patient populations.

The Court ordered ratios for mental health workers led to staffing levels for this group of employees that were among the richest of any state system in the country, consuming a substantial portion of the Department's human resources budget. The Department was thus limited in its ability to hire other key treatment personnel such as registered nurses, psychiatric social workers, and psychiatrists whose numbers were not addressed by the Court ordered staffing ratios.

Is I have noted, I was disillusioned and distressed by this Court Order. Several Department officials, Dr. Gordy and I had presented reasoned and scientifically-based testimony agreeing in some areas with the Panel and disagreeing in others. Yet, the federal judge rejected all of our arguments and accepted in toto the claims, however specious, of the Review Panel. The Court endorsed the Panel's recommendations even when to do so meant that the Court had to disregard the plain meaning of the words in the Settlement Agreement.

Although the March 30, 1984 Court Order was a major turning point in the history of R.A.J., it did not end disagreements between the Panel and the Department. Critical reports continued to be issued by the Panel and ensuing Court Orders generally sided with the Panel against the Department. When the Department requested that it be permitted to achieve the newly ordered staffing ratios by reducing hospital censuses as well as adding new mental health workers, the Court approved. In doing so, however, the Court extended the scope of its authority to the state's community mental health programs.

A major dispute involved the insistence of the R.A.J. Panel that all state hospital patients be given an absolute right to refuse medication, regardless of their symptoms, behaviors, and legal commitment status. Thus the Department would have been forced to maintain refusing patients with active psychotic or physically assaultive behaviors indefinitely in the hospitals, while at the same time being required to meet other R.A.J. mandates including preserving of the rights of these patients and affording them thirty hours of active programming per week. This issue is one of the few in which the U.S. District Judge came down on the side of the state agency, permitting us to carry out an elaborate appeal and review procedure we had designed to accommodate patients who refused medications. My staff and I were grateful for this ruling for without it patient care and the morale of our treatment personnel would have suffered immensely.

As troubling to me as the sometimes arbitrary and inapt findings and recommendations of the Panel was the Panel's habit of courting the press. Panel members and the Plaintiff's attorney held press conferences and gave interviews critical of the Department, usually before the Department had time to respond officially to the latest Panel report or to address the issues in a Court hearing. The vast majority of state media attempted to provide balanced coverage, contacting me or staff members for our side of the story. On the other hand, a reporter for the only daily newspaper in the state capitol, Austin, was unceasingly hostile to the Department and me, providing a perfect vehicle for the Review Panel. Her news stories, really editorials in disguise, portrayed sympathetically the position of the Panel while ridiculing by means of factual distortions or selective quotations the responses of the Department. Since the reporter's articles were often picked up by wire services, her biased account of events frequently appeared in newspapers outside of Austin.

The press conferences and media contacts of the Panel and Plaintiff's attorney were troubling to the staff of the Department's facilities. The vast majority of employees working on state hospital wards respected the rights of patients in their care, were attentive to their needs, participated actively in their treatment, and would never harm or abuse them. They often told me of their anger and frustration upon reading newspaper accounts of the horrors that were alleged to take place in their work environments. Sensational news stories emanating from both the R.A.J. and Lelsz lawsuits increased in frequency to the point of crisis, resulting in a decline of staff morale throughout the entire system. By mid 1987, I felt compelled to write an open letter to all of our employees, expressing my appreciation and support for their work under difficult circumstances, explaining the source of the adverse publicity and placing the R.A.J. and Lelsz lawsuits in perspective.

My open letter, titled "Living Under Lawsuits,"[16] generated controversy as well a gratitude on the part of rank and file Department employees who had felt helpless as their jobs, their facilities, and their personal integrity were repeatedly assaulted by one-sided media coverage.

Because it conveys the emotional tenor of the times as well as my views of the lawsuits, especially their intrusion into day to day management of state facilities without the usual checks and balances that limit the power of ordinary managers, I shall quote the open letter in its entirety:

LIVING UNDER LAWSUITS

From: The Commissioner, Gary E. Miller, M.D.
To: ALL TXMHMR Employees
Date: July 1, 1987

This is a difficult time for TXMHMR employees. Almost daily the public is told by television, radio and newspapers that our department is doing a poor job in caring for people with mental illness and mental retardation.

I have no doubt that these media reports have led some people to think that TXMHMR employees do not care about their clients or that they lack the knowledge and skills necessary to provide quality services for them.

But what I fear most is that some of you may come to doubt the value of your work or of your services to our clients. The continuing publicity about allegedly poor care in our state hospitals and state schools cannot help but undermine the morale of the people who work for our department. The bad publicity and some other problems I will discuss later are what prompted me to write this special message to you.

The first point I want to make is that the stories in the press about poor care are either untrue or gross exaggerations. Except for isolated instances of abuse or neglect—which occur in every health care setting—the services you provide are not just "adequate"; they are exceptional. If objective measures were used to compare our MHMR programs to programs in other states and even some of those in the private sector, the Texas system would be ranked near the top. Our state facilities and community programs are at least the equal of most others; in many cases, they are much better. I am not arguing that our system is perfect or that it could not use more money and more staff. I am saying only that we do an excellent job with the money we have—in fact, a better job than a lot of other states that spend more money.

Some of the newspaper accounts of TXMHMR facilities must seem incredible to those of you who work daily on the dormitories and wards of those facilities—as they must seem incredible to the hundreds of visitors and volunteers who have intimate knowledge of the care you give to our clients. Unfortunately, less knowledgeable members of the general public may conclude from the media stories that our hospitals and schools are bad places. They may worry about what could happen if a family member is admitted to a TXMHMR facility; they may even fear for the safety of a relative or friend who resides in a facility.

Although the bad publicity is a serious problem for our department, our clients and the people of Texas, I believe we will eventually be able to tell the public about the fine job that you do. I am committed to using all available departmental resources to get that message across.

My second point is that most of the bad publicity can be traced to the two class-action lawsuits against the department (R.A.J. v. Miller and Lelsz v. Kavanagh). Although often sensational in tone, inaccurate and misleading, the publicity is not the fault of the press. The journalists who produce it are just doing their jobs. And as I have said, it is not your fault. You and your fellow employees do a good job under what are sometimes less than ideal conditions.

Why is it then that the professional judgments of our clinicians are assailed in public merely because some other "expert" has a different opinion? Why is it that our state hospitals are attacked in the press as substandard when (unlike those of most other large states) they all meet the only nationally recognized standard—accreditation by the Joint Commission on Accreditation of Hospitals? Why is it that we are subjected to media claims that the programs of our state schools are inadequate when they all comply with stringent federal Medicaid standards?

The answer, as I have suggested, lies with the two class-action lawsuits. The issue is not whether the plaintiffs were justified in filing the lawsuits in 1974 or even whether the lawsuits are, on balance, good or bad for the people we serve.

It is just that the lawsuits permit—or encourage—actions on the part of the participants that complicate our already formidable task of serving the state's mentally retarded and mentally ill.

The bad publicity is one of those complications, but there are others just as serious. Here are some detrimental effects of the lawsuits which, as you will see, include but extend beyond the problem of bad publicity.

The lawsuits violate basic management principles. The present structure of the lawsuits directly affects the administration of our department. It is easy to forget—because we usually think of lawsuits in terms of lawyers, courtrooms and black-robed judges—that lawsuits can take a managerial role, intruding into the agency's policy making authority and directing the work of its employees. That is what has been happening to TXMHMR since the R.A.J. and Lelsz lawsuits were settled in 1981 and 1983. (I use the word "settled" advisedly. Although technically the cases were settled when the parties negotiated Settlement Agreements that were later approved by the courts, the settlements marked the beginning rather than the end of intense adversarial activity.)

Let me explain how the lawsuits result in management decisions that violate basic management principles. Today, court appointed monitors (an expert consultant in Lelsz, a review panel in R.A.J.) inspect our department programs (often with the help of other experts they hire), form conclusions about the job we are doing and pass those conclusions on to the court and—as we have seen—to the media.

The monitors and their consultants are not the only experts who make pronouncements about the department. Other parties in the lawsuits (the plaintiffs who file the suits and several organizational intervenors) also send their experts to review our programs and announce their conclusions to the court and the public.

Sometimes these experts offer suggestions that can help us do a better job. Most of the time, their reports are critical of our work. Minor problems are exaggerated; isolated incidents are portrayed as typical of an entire state hospital or state school, or of all state hospitals or state schools; opinions of outside professionals which are usually no better than and sometimes not as good as those of our own TXMHMR professionals are presented to the courts and the public as the only "correct" or "acceptable" way of doing things.

Thus, we read in the newspaper that our programs are unacceptable, our professionals inadequately trained and our clients systematically abused and neglected.

All of this is frustrating to me as I know it is to you. We rarely have the opportunity to challenge or question the accuracy of the conclusions of these court monitors and experts. And on those rare occasions when we do have that opportunity, we are automatically on the defensive. Unlike the criminal justice system where one is presumed innocent until proven guilty, we are assumed to be guilty and must struggle to defend the care we provide to our clients.

Federal judges do not simply think about or study accusations made by our adversaries and our defenses against them; they act. The enormous power of the federal court is exercised in the form of court orders. We have been told in exquisite detail how many mentally retarded people from certain categories we were required to place from state schools into community programs in a year's time; we have been told how many mental health workers must be present on every ward of every state hospital; we have been told that community MHMR centers are now to be known as department facilities; we have been told that there is "too much" violence in our state hospitals, even though there was not a shred of evidence to support that conclusion. If we are told by a district court that red is blue, we have no choice but to accept the court's decision unless and until an appellate court reminds the district court that the color is really red.

Court orders thus affect the department's management of personnel, finances and treatment programs. Unlike normal management practices, these management decisions represent the exercise of power without accountability. You and I have superiors. We are given direction about what sort of work and accomplishments are expected of us. Our supervisors look at how we perform and hold us accountable for the results. Beyond those basics, as state employees we are responsible ultimately to the people of Texas. The elected representatives of the people — the governor, lieutenant governor and legislators — make state policy, write the laws and select the members of our state board who, in turn, direct my activities and yours.

This political constituency to which we in TXMHMR are accountable and the accountability that we all have within our agency are almost entirely lacking in the control of our department by the federal courts.

Anyone who is the least bit familiar with management principles knows that authority and responsibility must go together. That is clearly not the case in management by court order. The department is always the fall guy. If something goes wrong in our facilities, it is our fault; whatever progress is made is of course to the credit of the lawsuits and the court monitors. The court monitors can do no wrong; they do not have to account directly or indirectly to the people of Texas for the correctness of their conclusions about TXMHMR facilities or for the accuracy of their statements to the press.

The lawsuits violate another basic management principle: that decisions should be based on the best available information. A federal judge may be motivated to "reform" a state institution, but the structure of the lawsuits guarantees that the judge will have neither the information necessary to make good management decisions (that is, issue court orders) nor reliable information about how his decisions affect the state institution. Private conversations with court monitors, briefs filed by lawyers and legal rhetoric in the courtroom are simply not the equivalent of the comprehensive flow of accurate information and feedback that a manager would need in order to make important decisions about a complex program like a state hospital or state school.

For example, a manager with the authority to make decisions about such things as staffing and treatment programs in our facilities would normally not exercise that authority without first spending some time at the facilities and becoming familiar with your work by talking to you and your clients, learning something about what people with mental illness and mental retardation are like and learning as much as possible about treatment methods and their limitations. Obviously, none of this is possible under the peculiar management structure dictated by the lawsuits.

The real responsibility for care of the patients and clients rests with you and me, the employees of TXMHMR. Our job is not made any easier by the bad management practices that result from the lawsuits.

The Public Is Being Misled

This is where the bad publicity comes in. Let me begin by describing how I believe our adversaries view their role in the lawsuits. They are the good guys, out to reform an antiquated and inadequate system of care. We, on the other hand, are the defenders of the old and bad way of doing things. They are the people who really care about our clients; we are merely bureaucrats collecting our paychecks. It is they, not we, who are "concerned" about client abuse, good treatment planning and habilitation programs.

It is ironic that people like you who take on some of the most challenging and difficult jobs in government for relatively low pay are viewed as the problem by monitors and outside experts. Not only do you care, not only are you concerned about our patients and clients, it is you who have shown your willingness to do something about it. You made a personal commitment to help the patients and clients of this department by taking on a care and treatment or management and support role. Your role is vital to the well-being of our clients—and a lot tougher then standing on the sidelines and criticizing our facilities.

I began this section with a description of how I believe our adversaries view their role and ours. It is the structure of the lawsuits and the resulting poor management practices that permit these views of the monitors, plaintiffs and intervenors to be broadcast to the public as though they were proven facts. As we have seen, when there is no accountability—no reason to be accurate, to explain or to defend one's opinions—we have what is in effect an invitation to distort the facts.

Will the Lawsuits Ever Go Away?

TXMHMR employees must wonder whether our agency can ever do enough or be good enough to be released from the jurisdiction of the federal court.

I wish that getting out from under these lawsuits were simply a matter of doing everything the department said it would do in the Settlement Agreements in Lelsz and R.A.J.. Unfortunately, our experience in Texas and our knowledge of similar lawsuits in other states tells us that won't happen.

Both Lelsz and R.A.J. have demonstrated a tendency to create new issues on a regular basis, that is, to find new things wrong about what we do, thus expanding the scope of the lawsuits and the number of areas that must be monitored by the court. This serves, of course, to perpetuate the lawsuits, to keep them moving along from year to year like a runaway train.

It is not difficult to figure out the motivation of various parties for those activities that expand and continue the lawsuits. People seldom give up power voluntarily, especially when the power is exercised without accountability. There must be a good deal of gratification in exercising power over a state agency, summoning up vast quantities of indignation and concern about conditions in our facilities for the benefit of the press, and having no need to defend one's actions or take any political heat.

Economic forces are also at work. A lot of people make a lot of money as long as the lawsuits continue. There are attorneys' fees, expensive outside experts and of course the money that pays the salaries of the monitors and members of their organizations.

Although the court monitors are doubtless motivated by a desire to reform a state system they perceive as requiring reform, they also do this for a living. Their job depends on there being enough work for them to justify their continued employment. Thus, they have little motivation to find our department in compliance with various provisions of the Settlement Agreements and a lot of motivation to read new meanings into the language of those agreements and to discover new "problems" that raise compliance issues and require more monitoring.

The lawsuits seem as though they will drag on forever, but there are some things we can do to make them "go away."

What can we do?

We are not helpless. There are actions we are taking and can take that will ultimately lead to our vindication in the eyes of the public and to resolution of the lawsuits.

First, it is important that you continue to do the good job you are doing. It is easy to become distracted or discouraged because of the bad publicity and other pressures of the lawsuits. Nevertheless, we must work as hard as we can at our various jobs to keep up the quality of care we give to our patients and clients and to efficiently administer our agency and its facilities.

Second, we must continually improve our delivery system and the treatment of people in our care. This means, among other things, working with the governor and the legislature to increase our funding (already being done), keeping up to date with modern techniques through training and continuing education, improving the individual program and treatment planning for our clients and patients, and striving to improve our management of personnel and other resources of the department.

Third, we must get the message to the people of Texas that we do a good job in serving the mentally retarded and mentally ill, and that our treatment programs are constantly improving. The department will initiate an intensified public information program which will involve Central Office and all of our facilities. You will hear more about this later.

Finally, we must deal with the lawsuits on their own terms, that is we must vigorously defend the interests of our agency and the state of Texas in the federal courts. I am extremely pleased with the staff of the Attorney General's Office who represent our agency. They have done a superb job not only as articulate legal advocates for our department, but also as colleagues, supporters and even as advisors on ways to improve our programs.

The department won a decisive victory in January when the Fifth Circuit Court of Appeals overturned an order of the District Court and prohibited court-ordered quotas for community placement of mentally retarded people. The language of the Fifth Circuit opinion offers us hope that the lawsuits may eventually be resolved. For example, in discussing the plaintiffs' argument that a District court judge has the right to interpret a settlement agreement in any way he wants so long as the judge's orders are consistent with the spirit of the agreement, the Fifth Circuit said: "If, as appellees (plaintiffs) argue, a federal court may take almost any action against a state to enforce a consent decree (settlement agreement) so long as it is "consistent with" the "spirit" of the applicable constitutional law and the decree itself, there is no limitation on the scope of the court's power. Lack of restraint on an organ of government (even the judiciary) is the antithesis of law."

Let me end this message by reminding you how much I appreciate the contribution that each of you makes to this department. I am confident that the problems created by the lawsuits will eventually be a thing of the past. Our efforts can do a lot toward achieving that end.

Gary E. Miller, M.D.

Even under the best of circumstances, the job of a state mental health commissioner is difficult if not "impossible."[17] Intense political pressures, demands of multiple constituencies, often in conflict, and inevitable budgetary limitations make the commissioner's job one in which mere survival constitutes a degree of success. In Texas during the period of 1982-1988, the class action lawsuits, R.A.J. and Lelsz, added an additional, sometimes overwhelming, burden to the already difficult task I faced as commissioner.

Despite the unremitting pressures of the class action lawsuits, the staff of the Texas Department of Mental Health and Mental Retardation performed admirably during this period. Measurable gains were made in virtually every aspect of the state mental health-mental retardation system.[18, 19] Many of these improvements resulted from the dedication and diligence of employees in the agency's central office, state facilities and community programs. Some improvements were creative responses to lawsuit demands.

Separate divisions relating to institutions and community mental health-mental retardation programs were abolished in a major reorganization in July 1982 which led to administrative integration of state hospitals and community mental health programs.[20]

In 1982, the department, on its own initiative, established the Client Services and Rights Protection office to investigate instances of patient abuse or denial of patients rights. The Office monitored and enforced state laws, department rules and R.A.J. requirements relating to the rights of patients in all settings.

In 1983, a single point accountability system was established with designation of 63 local mental health authorities responsible for care of people with mental illnesses in each of 63 local service areas. In the same year, for the first time in its history, the department conducted site reviews of community mental health and mental retardation programs to assess the quality of their services and the degree of their coordination with state facilities.[21, 22] 1983 also saw the development of a statewide case management system that led to proactive and personalized care of thousands of people with severe and disabling mental illnesses.[23, 24, 25]

The department responded to the court order in R.A.J. requiring staff to patient ratios by developing a novel fiscal incentive system to reward community programs for reducing their use of state hospitals.[26, 27] This program and a counterpart for people with mental retardation (Prospective Payment System) anticipated the rapid growth of managed care in private sector health services.

These and many other improvements throughout the state mental health system were made without substantial budget increases, but were the result of innovative and efficient management of resources already available to the department. By 1988, the department had achieved a dramatic reduction of state hospital censuses, a drop in hospital recidivism rates, an increase in the volume of mental health services being provided in communities and a significant shift of funding from state hospitals to community programs.[18, 19]

It is not possible to identify or quantify benefits of the R.A.J. lawsuit to Texas' mental health system and the people it serves. The themes of R.A.J.—institutional reform, protection of patient rights and expansion of community alternatives—were themes already embraced by me, the state agency, and, for that matter, the mental health agencies of virtually every other state.[28, 29] There is no way to rewind and replay the tape to determine what would have become of the Texas mental health system in the absence of R.A.J. The agency has continued to improve services to its patients. R.A.J. has been "resettled" several times, most notably with a new settlement agreement in 1992, and the lawsuit—23 years old at this writing—trudges on but seems to be winding down.

On balance, it must be said that R.A.J. called attention to deficiencies in the state mental health system and helped to educate the state legislature and public about these deficiencies. It may have indirectly helped the department in its efforts to obtain increased funding and budgetary flexibility. It created a climate that made possible innovative programs such as the fiscal incentive system for diverting patients from state hospitals.

As one who lived through six years of turmoil generated by R.A.J. (and Lelsz) and bore the brunt of the adverse publicity and political problems caused by the class action lawsuits, my attitude toward R.A.J. is, for the most part, negative. That being said, I end this chapter by observing that what has happened has happened; we cannot change history. Oversight by the federal court will end, a prospect that I know will bring considerable relief to my successors now in charge of the department. They will be left with all of the ordinary demands, problems and controversy that accompany the task of running a massive state mental health department for the benefit of its patients.

References

1. Texas Department of Mental Health and Mental Retardation 1969 Annual Report. Austin, Texas, Texas Department of Mental Health and Mental Retardation, 1969.

2. Texas Department of Mental Health and Mental Retardation: Rules, regulations and standards governing the provision of mental health and mental retardation services by boards of trustees operating a community center or centers. Austin, Texas, Texas Department of Mental Health and Mental Retardation, 1969.

3. Miller, G.E.; "The Unit System: A New Approach in State Hospital Care," Texas Medicine, 65:44–51, 1969.

4. Miller, G.E.; Goldberg, L.; "Toward a Single System of Mental Health Services." Presented to Southwestern Regional meeting, the American Orthopsychiatric Association, Galveston, Texas, November 1972.

5. Miller, G.E.; Personal Advocacy in Action: Department of Human Resources, Division of Mental Health, Personal Advocacy Unit. Atlanta, Georgia, Division of mental Health, Georgia Department of Human Resources, October 1, 1973.

6. Seabrook, C.; "Mental Patients' Gripes Aired: State Complaints Now Met Head-On," Atlanta, Georgia, Atlanta Journal, December 4, 1973, p. 2c.

7. Miller, G.E.; Guidelines on Institutional Participation in Community Mental Health Programs. Atlanta, Georgia, Georgia Department of Human Resources, Division of Mental Health, January 1974.

8. Miller, G.E.; New Directions in Mental Health. Exploring Mental Health Parameters, F.R. Crawford, ed., Atlanta, Georgia, Paje Publishing Co., July 1974, pp. 57–60.

9. Gay, R.D.; "The Georgia Experience: Another Perspective. Unified Mental Health Systems: Utopia Unrealized, New Directions in Mental Health Services, #18," J.A. Talbott, ed., New York, Jossey-Bass, June 1983, pp. 67–71.

10. "Open Hospital Sparks Controversy: Feud Erupts Between Senator Culver Kidd and Dr. Gary Miller," Milledgeville, Georgia, The Union Recorder, October 11, 1973, p. 1.

11. Lee, D.; "Sexual Fears Dominate 'Open Hospital' Debate: Carter Blames Kidd for Hospital Controversy," Macon Georgia, Macon News, October 19, 1993, p. 1a.

12. Nordan, D.; "Carter Says Kidd Preys on Patients: Political Game?," Atlanta, Georgia, Atlanta Journal, October 19, 1973, p. 1a.

13. Miller, G.E.; "New Hampshire's Transition, in VI. Reorienting State Policy and Planning. A Network for Caring: The Community Support Program of the National Institute of Mental Health," Boston, MA, Center for Rehabilitation, Research and Training in Mental Health, 1983, pp. 56–62.

14. Ferriter, T.; "Dr. Miller: Put Resources Where People Are," Concord, New Hampshire, Concord Monitor, December 14, 1977, p. 1.

15. R.A.J. v. Miller, Memorandum Opinion and Order, March 30, 1984.

16. Miller, G.E., "Living Under Lawsuits," Memorandum to all employees of the Texas Department of Mental Health and Mental Retardation, Austin, Texas, Texas Department of Mental Health and Mental Retardation, July 1, 1987.

17. Miller, G.E., Iscoe, I.; A State Mental Health Commissioner and the Politics of Mental Illness. Impossible Jobs in Public Management, E.C. Hargrove, J.C. Glidwell, ed., University Press of Kansas, 1990, pp. 103–132.

18. Miller, G.E.; "Progress Report, Texas Department of Mental Health and Mental Retardation," Austin, TX, Texas Department of Mental Health and Mental Retardation, January 18, 1985.

19. Miller, G.E.; "TXMHMR: A Retrospective," address presented at meeting of the Hogg Foundation for Mental Health, Austin, TX, January 22, 1988.

20. Miller, G.E.; "Reorganization," Memorandum to Chairman and Members of the Texas Board of Mental Health and Mental Retardation, Austin, TX, Texas Department of Mental Health and Mental Retardation, April 2, 1982.

21. Miller, G.E.; "TDMHMR Community Standards for Community Mental Health and Mental Retardation Centers and Community Service Programs of TDMHMR," Austin, TX, Texas Department of Mental Health and Mental Retardation, May 1995.

22. Miller, G.E.; "Establishment of TDMHMR Evaluation Component," Austin, TX, Texas Department of Mental Health and Mental Retardation, November 3, 1983.

23. Miller, G.E.; "Case Management Manpower Taskforce," Austin, TX, Texas Department of Mental Health and Mental Retardation, April 14, 1983.

24. "Case Managers are Guardian Angels in Human Service," Impact, XII:5, Austin, TX, Texas Department of Mental Health and mental Retardation, March–April 1983, pp. 10–12.

25. Miller, G.E.; Case Management: The Essential Service. Case management in Mental Health Services, C. J. Sanborn, ed., New York, Haworth Press, 1983, pp. 3–15.

26. Miller, G.E., Rago, W.V.; "Fiscal Incentives to Development of Services in the Community," Hospital and Community Psychiatry, June 1983, 39:6:595–597.

27. Fincannon, J.; "Staff-to-Patient Ratios in State Hospitals," Austin, TX, Texas Department of Mental Health and Mental Retardation, July 23, 1984.

28. Ahr, P., Holcomb, W.R.; "State Mental Health Director's Priorities for Mental Health Care," Hospital and Community Psychiatry, 1985, 35:39–45.

29. Miller, G.E.; "Program and Policy Issues of State Government, in II. Perspectives from the State Level. A Network of Caring: The Community Support Program of the National Institute of Mental Health," Boston, MA, Center for Rehabilitation, Research and Training in Mental Health, 1985, pp. 7–13.

Chapter 6

The Positive Impact of R.A.J.

Don Gilbert

Most state mental health commissioners will concede that a major class action lawsuit thankfully brings a measure of positive reform along with the inevitable grief and embarrassment. The federal court commands the attention of the legislative and executive branches of state government like nothing else can. At the heart of most reforms— more and better trained staff, improved quality of care, recognition of patient rights, among others—is the reality of increased funding.

In Texas, there is little argument that the R.A.J. class action lawsuit has been the primary influence in the expansion of mental health funding. The following chart reflects the growth of mental health funding between 1977 when early settlements were negotiated and 1993 when the final settlement agreement was reached.

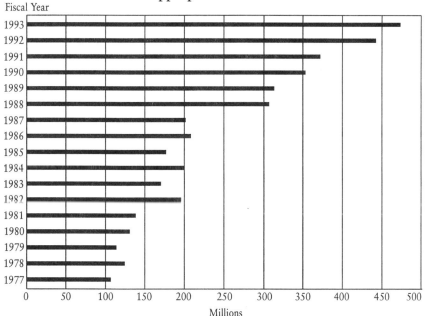

At first, the additional appropriations came with relative ease. The considerable media coverage depicting the inadequacies of the state hospital system forced elected officials to recognize that conditions in the state hospitals had to improve. The 1981 Settlement Agreement offered legislators the hope that compliance and final resolution to the lawsuit was within reach and the purse strings loosened. The lawsuit persisted, however, and the frustrations of both the legislature and the executive branch were evident. Budget hearings often found the department making feeble excuses about its lack of compliance with the settlement agreement while the federal court monitor attempted to explain to legislative leaders that increased appropriations were absolutely imperative lest the wrath of the federal court be brought to bear. "Forced funding" under the veiled and not so veiled threats of the federal court became a source of great irritation for legislators. With each biennial legislative session came the expectation that additional funding would lead to settlement of the lawsuit, however, each new biennium found either new interpretations of need or a lack of progress in state hospital reform.

Increased funding, however, has not been the only advantage to result from the R.A.J. lawsuit. Real improvement in the quality of care has been evidenced throughout the state hospitals in Texas. It's difficult to judge how much of the improvement in care is attributable to the lawsuit, as no doubt progress would have occurred regardless of the oversight from the federal court. It is widely agreed that the great majority of the reform in state hospital care has been the direct result of court monitoring and the additional resources that followed.

In retrospect, the care and treatment of individuals in Texas state hospitals in 1974 was atrocious, but at the time we didn't see it. At Terrell State Hospital just outside of Dallas, where the Jenkins (later R.A.J.) case originated, the 900 employees for the most part worked very hard to serve the needs of the nearly 2,000 patients residing there. The conditions in the hospital were unacceptable by today's standards, but in 1974 that was simply state hospital life. We were certainly aware of the crowding, the lack of privacy, and the chaotic environment, but within those constraints, staff worked with considerable caring to provide for men and women with mental illnesses. That caring was expressed in a paternalistic way with staff taking care of patients as a parent might take care of a child in need. The

The Positive Impact of R.A.J. 125

fact that the great majority of the staff were unskilled or at least untrained workers with very little in the way of professional supervision allowed well-intended but misguided approaches to care and treatment to abound. We didn't consider patient rights because, as a practical matter, state hospital patients at that time were guaranteed very little in the way of rights. The staff was in charge and the staff knew best. Psychiatric patients were not expected to participate in treatment decisions; that was the role of the staff. The role of the patient was to be compliant. While this approach to the care and treatment of mental illness is primitive by today's standard, it represented the paradigm for state hospital work in 1974.

The importance of this context is that while we can look back today with great indignation at those conditions and the practices, the sense of dedication and caring felt by the overwhelmed staff for the patients and the pride of work done well exemplified the attitudes of that period. Consequently, the filing of Jenkins v. Cowley in 1974 and its subsequent class action status as R.A.J. v. Gaver (and its ensuing designations under four successive commissioners as R.A.J. v. Kavanagh, R.A.J. v. Miller, R.A.J. v. Jones, and, finally, R.A.J. v. Gilbert) evoked feelings of hurt and humiliation on the part of both staff and the local community. There was the sense of having done the best you could to help patients and in return there was public ridicule and embarrassment.

Over the course of the next several years, Terrell State Hospital was virtually under siege from "expert observers" and plaintiffs' attorneys with production demands that kept the photocopiers working 24-hours-a-day. The media maintained a near constant surveillance with story after story about the atrocities of state hospital care. It seemed as though every disgruntled former employee talked to the Dallas news media and conveyed still another sensational story. Not all of the coverage was accurate, but there was enough truth about conditions in state hospitals that it made an indelible impression in the public's perception. The coverage also influenced perceptions within the mental health community. Word quickly spread among professionals that working at Terrell exposed one to the potential of regular scrutiny on the nightly news or, at the very least, to hours of interrogatories related to the lawsuit. The recruitment and retention of quality staff was next to impossible. By now, the legislature had recognized the seriousness of the situation with the federal court and had increased funding significantly. The stigma of the lawsuit, however, made it difficult to spend the money on staff.

In time, the sensationalism of the class action lawsuit faded and the reality dawned that, for all of its nuisance value, the lawsuit did bring regular funding increases. State hospitals underwent facelifts and staffing levels began to approach reasonable levels. As conditions improved, pride slowly began to return to the work force. The news value of state hospital life dissipated as the sensational stories became harder to find. There was a period of growth and renewed focus in the late 1970s and early 1980s that produced some very positive results.

Perhaps as a result of our collective feeling of accomplishment, a sense of unrest developed over the ongoing intrusion of the federal court into hospital operations. There was a feeling that no matter how much we improved, it was never enough. The apparent arbitrariness of the lawsuit irritated the professional staff considerably. An interesting conflict evolved between our wanting to be free from the external intrusion while knowing that additional funding depended on the federal court's ongoing dissatisfaction with our work. One memorable event illustrates this conflict. A discussion during a regular meeting of the TXMHMR board in Austin touched on the subject of staffing ratios for state hospitals. The parties had never agree on the appropriate levels of staffing and no objective data existed to instruct either the plaintiffs or the defendants. The issue had not been the principle point of the discussion, but somehow in the course of the exchange, a board member asked a staff level administrator what he thought a reasonable ratio of staff to patients should be at a state hospital. After some head scratching and sputtering around, the staffer allowed as how he thought that 1:5 was about right. This staffing ratio became the standard in the R.A.J. lawsuit. Plaintiffs' attorneys and the court monitor argued that the department by its own admission had stipulated the appropriate staffing pattern for state hospitals. The implementation of this staffing pattern, among other things, required additional resources. Lots of them. The legislature swallowed hard and appropriated the money, believing this to signal the end of the additional resource issue.

Allocating the money for compliance with the staffing ratios resulted in windfalls for many of the hospitals, which was met with wild approval by hospital staff and administrators. Operationalizing the staffing ratios, however, became a nightmare. Because the battle for a designated staffing ratio was hard fought, the plaintiffs' attorneys were not about to yield on implementation. For example, there were several ways to interpret the staffing ratios. On a ward by ward basis, 1:5 meant that for every ward (patient living area) of roughly 25 patients, there had to be a ratio of one staff person for every five patients. If the interpretation, however, applied the ratio to a typical hospital unit comprising several wards then the hospital had some flexibility to move staff within the unit to match acuity levels. Still another interpretation could be that the hospital in total must achieve the prescribed ratio, offering still more flexibility for nursing administrators to move staff to areas of greatest need. The early interpretations by the plaintiffs' attorneys were the most narrow, demanding that the ratio be met on a ward by ward basis. Reporting at this level of detail on a shift by shift basis was onerous.

Another set of issues related to the staffing ratios concerned which staff were counted. The department argued unsuccessfully that all staff should be included—nurses, LVNs, social workers, psychologists, etc. The narrower view of the plaintiffs' attorneys was predictably that the ratio only applied to direct care aide staff, and that the ratio referred to on-duty staffing, not, as we had assumed, to positions assigned for coverage. In other words if five staff were assigned to the morning shift for a ward with 25 patients in residence, the ratio would not be met if one of the five staff failed to show up for work. This created enormous problems for hospital staffing and even greater problems for the budget. The appropriation from the legislature assumed only enough salary dollars to budget for the prescribed ratios, not to cover an on-duty ratio. Consequently, since the ratio had to do with aide-level positions, and no such requirements extended to other essential hospital staff, hospitals were forced to shift from professional positions to aide-level staff. The unintended consequence was the ultimate sacrifice of scarce professional staff for the more immediate lawsuit-related need to meet ratios. Eventually a reasonable compromise developed that offered greater flexibility in staffing for patient acuity with appropriately trained personnel. However, over the course of the years, before this compromise was struck, countless dollars were misdirected and frustrations heightened.

In the early 1980s, a court-ordered panel consisting of a psychiatrist, an attorney, and a social worker who doubled as the coordinator of the panel began to visit the eight state hospitals. Initially, compliance reviews were conducted with little staff interaction; the panel members first would tour the hospital then sequester themselves for a private reading of countless records. It was never clear in those early days just what the panel members were hoping to find. Clearly, however, "it" was never found. The reviews typically lasted for three or four days and culminated in an exit conference of sorts in which the panel offered a mixture of generalizations about the meager progress since the previous review and stern admonitions to work harder and do better. No doubt the message from the panel was clearer than I recall, but the findings were never specific enough for staff to rebut or attempt to clarify, which lent itself easily to our dismissal of the review as biased and purely a function of surveyor style and preference.

The Review Panel gave way in time to only the Court Monitor and a group of consultants. In place of the psychiatrist and lawyer from the panel, we experienced out-of-state psychiatrists who served as regular consultants to the court monitor. The newly configured review process posed its own set of challenges. The vagaries of the previous panel were replaced in many cases with outright disagreement between the hospitals' medical/professional staff and the consultants. While the consultants possessed impressive credentials, they were in some instances unfamiliar with psychiatric practice in institutional settings, or at least in Texas institutional settings. Considerable acrimony developed between some members of the state hospital system and these consultants that at times tended to seem argumentative and personalized. When this occurred, the review process was compromised and lacked value to the clinical and administrative staff of the hospitals.

I recall the terrible tension that would begin to pervade Terrell State Hospital about a month before each scheduled review; I had been named superintended there in 1983. Believing that an adversarial attitude never serves the process or the outcome well, I would try to prepare the clinical staff for the review with carefully chosen words of encouragement and perspective. Before each review, the executive staff would strategize on a positive presentation of the progress we believed had been made. The opening sessions of these reviews would typically start with my presentation of a positive overview of the hospital's performance and improvement since the last review. The review would continue on an optimistic note that lasted about as long as it took for the consultants to sit down with a staff psychiatrist and treatment team to review their records. Invariably, the randomly selected records would contain some egregious omission or commission that prompted defensiveness and argument between the attending psychiatrist and the consultant. No matter how indefensible the finding, staff was obsessed with offering an explanation. This lead the consultants to become frustrated, then assertive and finally, in the minds of some, pompous and righteous in their determinations. Arguably, this made it more difficult for the consultant to give staff the benefit of the doubt on other matters as the review progressed. At the end of the three and sometimes four days of review, I was left with an angry and insulted medical/clinical staff struggling through an exit conference with the consultants who were by all rights ready to get home and not eager to return.

One of the greatest frustrations for me as a hospital superintendent was the lack of specificity in the settlement agreement. The lack of clear expectation in the settlement gave license to the court monitor and his consultants to interpret compliance as they went along. I'm sure that each of the consultants had a clear sense of what constituted adequate evidence of good medical care or individualized treatment planning, but those measures were never particularly clear to me or the medical/clinical staff. I'm not sure there was consistency across consultants either. We were left with the unmistakable sense that compliance would be an ever changing target on many of the lawsuit issues, and that only the consultants would know compliance when and if they found it. This approach to institutional reform was like pushing on a string; it was impossible to sustain momentum. The unfortunate element, in looking back, is that the department clearly had a long way to go towards providing adequate care for the men and women residing in its state hospitals. Both the process and the frustration of depending on the consultant to decipher the code for compliance caused many staff to discount the need to improve. The belief of most staff and administrators was that no matter how much better the hospitals performed, the bar over which we were expected to jump would continue to be raised. We lost sight of the important things in state hospital work and became preoccupied with illusive, external measures of satisfactory performance as judged by a group of consultants who came around every nine months or so to look at some records. Things had to change.

Over the years, I developed a good relationship with the court monitor and his consultants despite the frustrations of the process. I respected their expertise and perspectives even though I sometimes saw things differently. It was this comfort and trust which allowed me one evening over dinner to share with them what I thought might be the solution to lawsuit compliance.

It was 1989, and I was doing double duty, serving as the superintendent at Terrell and also as acting superintendent at Vernon State Hospital some 300 miles away. There had been significant staff turnover at the Vernon State Hospital as well as some pretty serious performance problems, and I was asked to split my time between the two facilities until a suitable replacement could be found for Vernon. During one of my stays at Vernon, the court monitor and his consultants arrived for a review. Over dinner their first night, we talked about how the lawsuit might conclude. My contention was that compliance would be an almost random event, related more to the chance finding of a good set of records than to the systematic demonstration of improved performance. I suggested that true systemic improvement relative to the lawsuit compliance issues would come only with each hospital's ownership of performance and internal improvement through measurement. Rather than looking for that magic point in time when just the right records would be pulled, we should be looking for a system that held each hospital accountable for maintaining a performance measurement system that focused on the issues of the lawsuit. External compliance reviews should concentrate on the adequacy of the internal system which in time would lead to the validation that a sustained level of care had been achieved throughout the hospital, not just in a one-time sample on a lucky day. This, of course, required a level of performance specificity that did not then exist. I believe this discussion set the stage for the settlement talks that would take place more than a year later.

In 1990, I moved to the department's Central Office as the acting deputy commissioner for mental health services; I had responsibility for the state hospitals as well as community-based mental health programs. As I look back on the beginning of the negotiation process for the 1991 settlement agreement, I am surprised that we were able to realize any progress. An enormous amount of acrimony had been rekindled between the department's Central Office, the plaintiffs' attorneys, and the court monitor. The fourteenth report to the court had just been released at the beginning of the 1991 biennial legislative session citing non-compliance and poor progress on most of the issues of the lawsuit. On the heels of that contentious report the department was about to propose a radical shift from court monitoring to self monitoring. We had been struggling with lawsuit compliance for a very long time, and the trust level among most of the players could not have been worse. Several things, however, were working in favor of resolution. First and, I believe, most importantly was the appointment of new plaintiffs' attorney, Ed Cloutman. Ed had the reputation of being very tough but also very reasonable. It was his reasonableness that kept the discussions alive on many occasions when many thought we had reached an impasse. The other factor working in favor of a new agreement was the fact that I had developed a relationship with the court monitor and his consultants that allowed me to be viewed as credible in the negotiation process. For the most part I enjoyed these consultants and, in fact, found them very interesting. They, in turn, viewed me not as a "Central Office" staffer there to fight with the parties but as a state hospital superintendent who had passed the test of competence with the court monitor and just happened to be in the dual role of acting deputy commissioner for mental health services and lead negotiator. The final point in favor of productive negotiation is that we had a decent approach to resolution at a time when practically everyone was worn out with the existing process of compliance monitoring.

I had long believed that the solution in R.A.J. was for the department to become proficient in the process of continuous quality improvement (CQI). If the administration and staff of state hospitals could first understand the expectations of R.A.J. and then create measurable performance improvement systems using CQI tools, it seemed reasonable that the department could demonstrate a level of sustained compliance that would put an end to the lawsuit. I had lost faith in the ability of the court monitor's consultants to independently see the kind of change that I believed the system was capable of achieving. The consultants, after all, had been doing battle with the medical/clinical staff of the eight state hospitals for years; it would be extremely difficult for them to enter a hospital they had reviewed a half dozen times or more without some level of bias. I wanted to find a way to return the evaluation of quality to its rightful place: with those actually involved in doing the work. What I lacked was a vehicle to assure that each hospital evaluated quality the same way. We had to be sure that each local system of quality improvement produced the same results. The answer came to me during a workshop conducted by the Motorola Corporation.

By mid-1990, the department was heavily into the learning phase of continuous quality improvement. A regular training feature for the commissioner's executive staff involved monthly presentations by private companies on their quality improvement efforts. Motorola Corporation, which has two manufacturing facilities in Austin, the capital of Texas and location of the department's Central Office, had recently won the Malcomb Baldridge National Quality Award which recognizes U.S. companies for leadership in quality. At Motorola, quality was assured by a two-phase process in which each local operation assumed the primary role in measuring quality based on a uniform system developed for all operations in the Motorola organization. Periodically, teams of Motorola employees from various parts of the country come in for a validation of the local operation's quality assessment. In other words, a group of people who do similar work within the Motorola organization come into a sister site, and review the work done by that site to assess and improve quality. In this system, there is tremendous opportunity for cross pollination of strategies for success. This system also guaranteed that each local operation followed the quality assessment and improvement system prescribed by Motorola headquarters.

I was taken by the idea of using the professionals within the state hospital system in conjunction with outside consultants to validate that each state hospital was objectively evaluating its own performance and utilizing the tools of continuous quality improvement to achieve performance improvements. I was fairly certain that we could design a quality improvement system for state hospitals that ultimately would address the outstanding issues in the R.A.J. lawsuit while pursuing the larger issues of continuous improvement in all aspects of hospital activity. It was important that the quality improvement system not be perceived by hospital staff as simply a lawsuit-related activity, but instead as a tool to move hospital performance to a higher level. The Motorola idea of having external validation teams from within the organization allowed for the assurance that each hospital would fairly and conscientiously evaluate its own performance. We went to work developing the initial design for a continuous quality improvement system complete with external validation teams. This was the beginning of the system that became known as quality system oversight (QSO).

Fortunately, I had access to highly motivated and conscientious professionals in the department's Central Office who were willing to play major roles in conceptualizing the QSO design, and in the subsequent elaboration that became the basis for the R.A.J. settlement agreement. Diane Faucher, R.N., and Bill Rago, Ph.D., were uniquely qualified to work on this project. Diane is a psychiatric nurse with a tremendous capacity for working through complicated and detailed issues. Her clinical skills and knowledge of the state hospital work processes were invaluable. Bill has an encyclopedic understanding of continuous quality improvement and the principles of TQM, as well as an absolutely incredible mind. Bill and I would brainstorm in my office for hours at a time. Several days later, he would reappear with pages and pages of elaborately detailed narrative, charts, and graphs fleshing out our CQI approach. His ability to take a rough concept and construct a thorough and meticulous design was invaluable as we worked the concept of QSO into a form that could be presented in the settlement negotiations. Bill is without exception the best I've ever seen at bringing a concept to life with a level of detail that is simply dazzling.

At the first settlement meeting, I observed a significant amount of skepticism as we presented the outline of QSO. A great deal of development had been done on the design of the QSO system but we presented only the rough idea of how it was expected to work. It was essential that we not appear too far in front in order to sell the notion of genuine collaboration involving all the parties in the lawsuit. Throughout the settlement negotiations we tried to stay far enough ahead of the process so that we could effectively lead the discussions to the conclusions that we preferred.

Our initial presentation of QSO met with a mixed response among the parties, which included Ed Cloutman, the new lead plaintiffs' attorney; Randy Chapman, John Heike, the plaintiffs' attorneys who had been on the case, Helen Brattin, the amicus from the Texas State Employees Union; and David Pharis, the R.A.J. court monitor. The attorneys who had been involved with the lawsuit for a number of years seemed to be ready to dismiss the concept from the outset; the level of trust necessary for them to believe that the department could seriously implement a self monitoring system leading to a resolution of the outstanding issues was simply out of reach. On the other hand, Ed wanted to hear us out, and on several occasions in that first meeting encouraged his team to withhold judgment until we had a chance to fully describe how this system might work. From the first settlement meeting, Ed distinguished himself as a person interested in finding solutions rather than continuing the unproductive fight that had dragged on for years. I don't recall exactly how that first settlement meeting ended, but I do remember feeling encouraged that we at least had a reasonable chance at being heard on the subject of self monitoring through QSO.

The settlement meetings that followed were at times difficult but seldom contentious. There was a relatively brief period of posturing among the attorneys, which yielded to the more productive exercise of finding and building on points of agreement. The interested parties in R.A.J. wanted the same thing: improvement in the care and treatment of persons in state hospitals. From that basic understanding, we tried to identify and build upon points of agreement. The parties saw things differently both in terms of degree and in some of the fine points of definition and approach, but on balance there were more things about which we could agree than disagree. The substantive issues were ones on which we found considerable agreement; where we would sometimes get snagged was on the finer points of process.

If we were to be successful in resolving the lawsuit issues, we had first to define the issues of compliance, then decide how we would objectively measure performance in each area of compliance, and, finally, agree on the measurable performance levels that would indicate compliance. Once the compliance issues were defined, the next several months of negotiation focused on the development of instruments that would be used to evaluate performance in each of the compliance areas of the lawsuit. The work of developing instruments for measuring clinical performance was extremely tedious; the instruments had to reflect good clinical practice in a number of very technical levels of care while being simple enough for easy application to a significant number of clinical records. The strength of the proposed QSO system was that it would be applied regularly to a significant number of hospital events that would yield an accurate profile of hospital performance. In that regard, the instrumentation of the system had to be manageable. With the assistance of the consultants brought in by the court monitor, who had been involved for some time with compliance reviews, and the input from several professional staff from state hospitals, the instruments began to take shape.

Once the instruments were developed, it was time to begin to talk about compliance. The conflicts that pertained to the instruments were usually related to clinical preference or interpretation and, as such, were relatively easy to resolve. The questions pertaining to compliance were much less clear. The perennial issue of how well does the system have to perform before it is determined that the constitutional guarantees related to the lawsuit were met, was once again the point of contention. It seemed to me that the steps that remained in reaching agreement in this settlement negotiation were likely to be difficult without some frame of reference. Central Office had done some preliminary testing of these instruments in our state hospitals so that we had some idea of current performance, but we believed it would not have been wise to introduce the results of that into the settlement discussions for fear that whatever our current level of performance, it would by definition be insufficient from the plaintiffs' perspective. Since we needed some sort of reality check on performance levels indicated by the application of these instruments, we proposed that we select four or five state hospitals across the country that we could all agree were, by reputation, good hospitals and, therefore, benchmarks of quality institutional care for persons with mental illness. We would arrange for an application of our new instruments on the records of these hospitals.

As it turns out, there was very little in the way of objective measurement of state hospital care across the country. We asked the court monitor to develop a list of potential hospital sites from which we would negotiate down to a list of four or five, based primarily on the ones to which we were able to gain access. The final list included one hospital in Colorado, two in North Carolina, one in Missouri, and one in Virginia. The selection was based primarily on rankings of state hospital systems published in the 1990 third edition of Care of the Seriously Mentally Ill. The publication is a joint effort of the Public Citizen Health Research Group and the National Alliance for the Mentally Ill, and is commonly referred to as the "Fuller Torrey report" after the medical doctor who took the lead in developing and publishing the rankings. We were able to access these hospitals and their records through the commissioners' offices in the respective states. In exchange for the access to clinical records, which also required considerable support from local medical records staff, we agreed to conduct training sessions for local staff on our QSO system. As we conducted these training activities there was considerable validation for the process of QSO, which reinforced our resolve to get this system started in Texas. While our teams of experts scored instruments using hospital records, Bill Rago and I conducted training sessions in the selected hospitals. The more we trained, the better we felt about QSO.

In applying our instruments to these test sites we discovered a great degree of variability. Even though our benchmark hospitals were, according to the Fuller Torrey reports and other indicators, among the better state institutions across the country, our instruments suggested that some of these hospitals were much lower performers than others. As indicated earlier, we had done enough sampling in Texas to give me some assurance that our hospitals were not far off the performance levels of these benchmark hospitals. There was considerable value to our testing these instruments outside the State of Texas. First, I think that the R.A.J. consultants who had looked so critically at Texas hospitals for so many years gained a new perspective as they looked critically at these out-of-state, benchmark hospitals. They never specifically indicated this, but I think they saw that at least some of the Texas hospitals were already as good as these that had been established as benchmarks for the country. The other value was in our traveling together, working on this test project together, and having the opportunity to share opinions and observations outside of the often adversarial atmosphere of the site visits in Texas. I look back at the out-of-state trips we took in preparation for the final discussions on performance levels for lawsuit compliance as both a wonderfully interesting time and a very strategic effort to set the stage for settling on compliance levels.

Our position was that we had been to the "best" hospitals in the country, according to the court monitor and consultants, and surely the scores of these hospitals represented a higher level of performance than should be necessary to satisfy the conditions of the lawsuit. The court monitor and the plaintiffs tried to dismiss the poor performance at some of the test sites, but it was hard to deny with these instruments that we all agreed would test for the adequacy of medical care, individualized treatment, and other areas of patient care. We had used these instruments at hospitals that were by all accounts among the better hospitals in the country and gathered their performance for the purpose of negotiating performance levels. Ultimately, we would arrive at performance levels that represented a fairly high level of care, probably beyond that which would be considered by many people to represent the minimal constitutional guarantee for persons in psychiatric hospitals. I was comfortable with these levels; I believed they were achievable and represented a reasonable level of care. I also very much wanted QSO to be a system that pushed us toward continuous improvement. We were in the formative stages of applying the principles of TQM in the agency, and the idea of setting performance targets was already against the TQM grain. Setting them at what seemed a low level, say 65% or 70%, would clearly send the wrong message to the hospital system.

Implementation of the QSO model was a complicated process in many ways. The relationship between the department's hospitals and its Central Office had long entailed a great degree of autonomy, with each of hospital allowed to take its own course towards meeting the department's mission. The department had talked a lot about the entrepreneurial spirit, innovation, and empowerment. This was interpreted by many to mean that the hospital was free to do as it pleased in the areas of organization, resource deployment, and the pursuit of quality. The QSO system would require a great degree of uniformity among the eight state hospitals. We could not afford the variability that had been allowed, even encouraged, to exist. In order to demonstrate the department's ability to conscientiously and effectively evaluate the quality and appropriateness of services, there would have to be a single approach to defining, evaluating, and, to a large degree, improving quality. This was to be a significant leadership challenge. It should be noted that I was preparing to leave Central Office at about this time. My stint as acting deputy commissioner had been an interim appointment from the beginning. By statute, the mental health deputy in Texas must be a psychiatrist. I had occupied that office for almost a year at this point, and was committed to doing the first round of introduction and training on QSO with each of the eight hospitals before leaving.

Our training team who had been instrumental in the development of the QSO design and instrumentation, included Diane Faucher, Bill Rago, and the QSO coordinator, Doug Hancock. While it was impossible to totally separate QSO from the lawsuit, it was our hope that QSO would be seen as an integral system for sustained improvement in the quality of services at each hospital. Far more than instruments and compliance, QSO incorporated the principles of continuous quality improvement into the routine of state hospital operations. While the instruments initially focused on lawsuit related issues, the process, which included an elaborate hierarchy of interlocking teams, could easily expand to cover other hospital activities and system-wide concerns. In retrospect, I wish the issues originally covered in QSO could have been expanded to include some system concerns unrelated to the lawsuit, as selling QSO as a sustaining system for continuous improvement would have been much easier.

In the minds of the TQM/CQI purists, the department had prostituted the concept of quality. For them, we had lost the concept of the customer. We were attending to the external forces of the lawsuit, pursuing their definition of quality at the expense of the true customers—the persons receiving services and their family members. While it wasn't entirely true that we were ignoring the true customer in our definition and pursuit of quality, it was a fact that the definition of quality that we had built into QSO via the instruments and the performance targets was primarily driven by our settlement negotiations. I rationalized all of this by saying that the plaintiffs in this case were a certified class of individuals who receive services in our state hospitals (our true customers), and that the interests of our customers were being represented by their attorney, Ed Cloutman. It was on their behalf that he was bringing forth their definition of customer requirements, i.e., quality. This was a stretch for some, but I believed it to be a reasonable way of understanding the requirements in the context of pursuing quality as defined by the customer. It was also critical to the QSO process that our local team structure as well as the oversight team for the agency include customers—people who had experienced mental illness either personally, or through an immediate family member. These people added a richness and depth to the QSO process that was immeasurable.

The reaction to the initial rollout and training on QSO was mixed but generally positive. There had been considerable involvement of state hospital staff along the way, so the concept for at least some of the staff was not completely new. The early drafts of the instruments had been piloted in the hospitals, and the hospital leadership had been routinely briefed on the development of QSO. An extensive training manual was developed for the rollout and the training team was well prepared. The training covered an entire day, beginning with an overview of QSO and quality improvement, moving into the tools of quality improvement that would be necessary to effectively implement QSO, and followed by a review of the instruments of QSO and their use. There was considerable time allotted to practical exercises to give participants a hands on experience with the tools and instruments of QSO. The participants were generally the hospital clinical leadership, quality assurance staff, and key administrators.

Our first training session was at Terrell where I had been superintendent for several years prior to assuming the role of acting deputy commissioner for mental health services. We started there because the staff was believed to be the most forgiving audience. I also had a great many close associates at Terrell who would be supportive. The training team learned a great deal from the experience. While the material was well received, we found that it was considerably more complicated to present than we had anticipated. The staff was patient with our awkwardness and offered constructive advice for future further training.

The quality of the training improved as we moved across the state. As we completed a few training sessions, it became clear that some hospitals were going to do better with QSO than others. The acceptance of the training material and the QSO process was largely influenced by the attitude of the hospital leadership. Some hospital superintendents and clinical directors fully embraced the value of QSO and its focus on measurability and teams, while some were fairly indifferent. The staff's responsiveness and willingness to actively participate followed along these lines. I remember meeting active defiance of the QSO process and related training at only one hospital, manifested as a pronounced sentiment that QSO was a burden on an already overburdened staff and that the true measure of quality was more a function of clinical intuition and professional competence than measurements of what is in a chart. The challenge was polite and professionally delivered but highly frustrating. This was the only training experience from which the team left with the feeling that our efforts were not productive. As we completed the training at the eight state hospitals, we compared predictions about the success of each of the hospitals with regard to QSO performance. While the team differed slightly on which hospitals might be the first to exit the lawsuit through the QSO process, there was the unanimous feeling that the one hospital where the leadership had resisted the QSO training would be the last to show improvement. That has proven to be true, although with a change in leadership and a commitment from the top in the QSO process, that hospital has shown remarkable progress in the last year or so.

As I write this, I've served for two and one-half years as the commissioner of the Texas Department of Mental Health and Mental Retardation. I am now able to look back on the development of QSO from a different perspective. QSO has evolved over the past five years and has been incorporated into the fabric of state hospital activity. There is no doubt that QSO has improved the quality of service in our state hospitals, probably in a profound way. At the time of this writing, all but one of the eight state hospitals have fully exited the lawsuit. The remaining hospital is only months away from satisfying the final requirements. All of the hospitals that have exited the lawsuit have done so since I have been in the job of commissioner, which has afforded me the opportunity to celebrate the accomplishment with those hospitals. QSO, of course, continues at those hospitals, as designed.

I think that the most reinforcing moment for me in all of my experience with QSO came about a year ago when one of our hospitals was dismissed from the lawsuit. The superintendent of that hospital is a close friend, and when I received the news about the success, I was excited and enthusiastic about calling him to offer my congratulations. I was taken aback by his lack of exuberance over the situation. He explained that while he and his staff understood why the rest of the Department was pleased and excited to have one more hospital on the verge of exiting the lawsuit, for them QSO had nothing to do with a lawsuit or even with compliance levels; QSO was simply the way they did their business, a reading on quality. And while there were obviously some thresholds of quality that had some significance to them and the rest of the system, passing those thresholds signified improvement, not accomplishment. That is the commitment to quality that we hoped to see with quality system oversight.

Chapter 7

Measurement of Psychiatric Care

David Pharis and Douglas Heinrichs

The 1981 Settlement Agreement required that all patients should have the right to individualized treatment planning by qualified mental health professionals. Each treatment plan should fully describe the patient's diagnosis, specific problems, and specific needs, and a description of short and long term goals and time frames for their attainment. Patients should have the right to have sufficient staff available to provide adequate individualized treatment, planning, and programming.[1]

The concept of individualized treatment was not defined further by the Settlement Agreement. However, TXMHMR facilities were meeting JCAHO standards which defined treatment planning and the Defendants had further defined treatment planning by its requirements for the patient record.[2] In 1981 TXMHMR was using a problem-oriented record system. This system was consistent with current JCAHO requirements, which asked for assessments of problems, statements of goals and objectives, treatment strategies to meet those goals, and reassessment to see whether the patient was making progress. It was also consistent with one of the few texts on the topic available at that time.[3] Although allegations of inadequate treatment had been made by experts in the discovery phase of the case, there may have been some expectations by the parties and the Review Panel that the concept of individualized treatment was understood in the same way by all.

When the Review Panel first looked at individualized treatment it familiarized itself with the Department's record system and asked

---

1. R.A.J. v. Miller, Settlement Agreement, 1981, p. 10.

2. Joint Commission on Accreditation of Hospitals, *Consolidated Standards Manual*, Chicago, IL, 1981, p. 61–81.

3. Brands, A. B., ed., *Individualized Treatment Planning for Psychiatric Patients*, Health Standards and Quality Bureau and the National Institute of Mental Health, Rockville, MD, 1982, p. 7–23.

questions of unit personnel about what they were wanting to accomplish with patients. Program descriptions were reviewed with the assumption that the Panel should accept statements about what the hospitals were attempting to do with patients, and then make clinical judgments concerning adequacy. The Panel assumed that multidimensional assessments would examine the biological, psychological, and social components of a person's illness and that each discipline would make specific contributions to treatment. The Panel expected that the treatment teams would develop an understanding of what brought a person into the hospital at a particular time and what would need to be accomplished to permit the patient to be discharged. The 1981 Consolidated Standards Manual from the JCAHO adequately defined assessment and treatment planning.[4] The Panel therefore assumed that since the record system was aimed at complying with JCAHO requirements that if staff used these guidelines that treatment would be adequate. During early reviews the Panel, however, concluded that treatment often was not individualized.

In the Second Report to the Court the Panel identified that many treatment plans were based upon problem descriptions that were too broad.[5] Several nonrelated issues were merged into one concept. For example, a patient's single problem was described as a psychological disturbance which included psychosis, confusion, paranoia, disorientation, and inappropriate affect. Such a multifaceted problem description defeated the goal of the problem identification process. Another shortcoming was the vagueness in the identification of problems. "Paranoia" is an example of a vague term that might refer to a very specific unrealistic fear.

Program activities often appeared to be based upon a formula. On one unit all patients were prescribed grooming to increase their self-esteem and everybody went to either the barber shop or beauty shop on a weekly basis. This strategy of grooming was prescribed to address a range of different problems for different patients. Although it is true that grooming may augment self-esteem it did not appear that

---

4. Joint Commission on Accreditation of Hospitals, *Consolidated Standards Manual*, Chicago, IL, 1981, p. 61–75.

5. R.A.J. v. Miller, R.A.J. Review Panel Second Report to the Court, May 1983, pp. 12–18.

all patients needed grooming as a therapeutic activity. Also, this approach elevated the barber or beauty shop to the level of a psychiatric intervention which did not seem to be appropriate.[6]

Another example related to a geriatric unit where all twenty patients were signed up for twenty-eight hours of toilet training a week.[7] The question was raised whether this was toilet training based on some kind of behavioral program or whether it was actually toileting. It turned out to be a toileting routine which raised the issue of the difference between therapeutic activities aimed at maintaining or increasing a person's functioning and routine nursing activities which are obviously necessary in such a facility.

By 1983 the Review Panel had developed a case record review instrument with twenty-two questions which gathered descriptive information from each of the records. This information included the Diagnostic and Statistical Manual (DSM) III diagnosis, current medications, dates of recent assessment for involuntary movements (AIMS) review, and specific descriptions from the treatment plan listing the goals, problem descriptions, and treatment strategies. Information was gathered about whether the patient had been involved in physical acting out behavior during the last forty-five days and whether such behavior was addressed as a problem in the treatment plan. The content of this instrument was based upon an understanding of JCAHO requirements. This instrument primarily gathered information from the treatment plan. There was no method for determining a score for the record. Conclusions therefore reflected the professional judgments of the reviewers.

During the years of implementation the Review Panel revised the clinical instruments several times through negotiations with the Defendants. Drafts were sent to the attorneys and program staff in central office and revisions were made which were used for data collection in the next round of reviews.

In 1986 an instrument was developed which began to collect judgments about the adequacy of treatment. The usual descriptive information was gathered about the DSM III diagnosis, the use of medica-

---

6. R.A.J. v. Miller, R.A.J. Review Panel Second Report to the Court, May 1983, p. 16.
7. R.A.J. v. Miller, R.A.J. Review Panel Tenth Report to the Court, July 1987, p. 15.

tions, the presence or absence of polypharmacy, and the screening for involuntary movements. Also, information was gathered about the number of program hours that a patient received each week. Then the following types of questions were asked:

- Are the reasons that a patient is unable to function in a community stated in the record?
- Is the treatment plan based upon problems identified in assessments?
- Are treatment goals which are relevant to improving the patient's capacity stated in the record?
- Are the relevance of the treatment strategies and intended benefits to the treatment goals stated in the record?
- Does the record reflect how the accomplishment of treatment objectives would be recognized?
- Does the record reflect that the treatment actions are being carried out?

Judgments were made about whether the question was answered "yes" or "no" or whether there was insufficient information to answer the question.

In 1987 this instrument was revised and expanded to include more questions about the process of treatment planning. Additional questions identified:

- Whether additional diagnostic evaluations were ordered when appropriate?
- Whether diagnoses were consistent with the current DSM manual?
- Whether all assessment data was considered appropriate when formulating the treatment plan?
- Whether termination criteria and discharge considerations were evident in treatment planning?
- Whether progress notes appropriately reflected prescribed treatments?
- Whether the responsible physician recorded clinical justification for medications prescribed and changes in medications?

- Whether there was clinical justification for special treatment procedures such as restraint and seclusion, ECT, and aversive therapy?

Again, judgments were made as to whether the questions should be answered "No," "insufficient information," or "Yes."

In 1990 this instrument was again revised and expanded through negotiations with the Court Monitor, his psychiatrist consultants, and the Defendants. The resulting instrument greatly expanded the amount of detail from which clinical judgments were made about the adequacy of care. A new scale was introduced for the determination of adequacy. The scale included judgments of better than adequate (BA), adequate (A), inadequate (I), very inadequate (VI), and not applicable (N/A). In terms of determining the adequacy of a psychiatric or social assessment the reviewer looked for descriptions of the present illness, past psychiatric history, drug and alcohol history, mental status, medical factors, family and social factors, occupation and educational factors, developmental history for child or adolescent, military history, legal history, and a summary of the above. The adequacy of nursing, physical, social, and activity assessments were reviewed as being required by the record system. Dietary, occupational, recreational, educational, psychological, dental, visual, and other medical consultations were all considered as optional assessments to be done as appropriate to the client situation. When special consultations were needed and done, they were reviewed for their adequacy. The question was raised about whether the case formulation was present from which a diagnosis and a treatment plan could be derived. Questions were then raised about the relevance of the treatment plans, goals, objectives, and interventions.

This questionnaire, which was detailed and comprehensive in its review of the treatment process, was also lengthy and cumbersome. The instrument contained twenty-four scoreable questions. However, these questions contained an additional thirty-seven scoreable items. All of these items could be scored in terms of adequacy, inadequacy, or being not applicable. This instrument was painstakingly revised and reviewed by the Defendants and was accepted by them prior to the Court Monitor's use of the instrument and data gathering for a major report to the Court.

However, before this document was somewhat accepted by the Defendants, issues about how and whether clinical care could be measured were aggressively argued. In July 1989, the Defendants objected vigorously to the use of the proposed clinical review instrument as an independent compliance measurement tool to measure the clinical issues of hospital care. The Defendants stated, "The process of evaluating individualized treatment, the sufficiency of programming and the proper administering of medication is inherently subjective." The document also stated, "The desire of the Court Monitor to replace these subjective reports with an objective, numerically scored compliance tool is desirable, but illusory. The scores will still reflect subjective opinions about the issues being evaluated. The importance of assuring a sound methodology in this instrument cannot be understated. If Defendants' compliance with individualized treatment and other issues is to be determined from the given hospital's score on this instrument, then the instrument must be consistent, accurate, and fair. Defendants are convinced that the instrument does not meet any of these tests."[8]

The Monitor challenged the Defendants' position that evaluating individualized treatment was inherently subjective. He argued that professional clinical judgment is based upon theory, knowledge, and experience in a particular field plus the ethical standards of the profession. Once professional expectations are made explicit it could be expected that there would be consistency among clinical judgments.

After the development of the QSO process and the establishment of the new 1992 Settlement Agreement, this instrument was revised again by the Monitor and Defendants to become the QSO instruments for individualized treatment, medication monitoring, and the use of special treatment procedures. The old instrument was divided into three separate instruments to deal with the cumbersome nature of the first instrument. At this point the Defendants accepted that the modified instruments measured consistently, accurately, and fairly.

During the implementation phase of this case, the question about what constituted individualized treatment was handled by the Monitor and the Defendants in at least two different ways. For the most part the issue was addressed through examining the treatment planning process as has been described above. The treatment was defined as containing assessments, diagnosis, formulation, treatment planning, treatment provision, and reassessment. The first iterations of

---

8. R.A.J. v. Jones, Defendant's Objection to Recommendation 71, July 1989.

treatment review were very descriptive in nature. Further reviews sometimes gave priority to specific details of the treatment planning process but also began to ask for judgments about the adequacy of the process. Although the Defendants repeatedly participated in these discussions, little true agreement was reached on these issues until the development of the QSO process and its incorporation in the 1992 Settlement Agreement. It may by that there was no incentive to reach agreements on the definitions of clinical care until there were decisions to reduce the adversarial relationships between the Parties and the Monitor. The Defendant's early reliance upon the adequacy of the professional judgment standard in Romeo v. Youngberg obviated the value to them of defining adequate clinical care.

In 1987 the Review Panel turned the focus of individualized treatment to the development of psychosocial programs for patients in the hospitals. In the Tenth Report to the Court the Review Panel concluded that the hospitals were not only out of compliance with the requirements for individualized treatment but that there were particular gaps of services in an area that could be called psychosocial programming.[9] The Review Panel, therefore, recommended that a nationally recognized consultant be asked to review the presence of psychosocial programming in the facilities and make recommendations for the further enhancement of such programming. In the negotiations that followed these recommendations, the Defendants did not agree with the Review Panel's findings of noncompliance but did accept the recommendation for consultation and training in the area of psychosocial programming. This different perspective about whether there was compliance or noncompliance in the area of treatment led the Review Panel, Defendants, and Plaintiffs to all have different expectations about whether assessments done by the psychosocial consultants could be used as a monitoring mechanism in the lawsuit. The Review Panel and Plaintiffs thought that the consultations could of course be used as continuing indicators of compliance. The Defendants adamantly maintained that, since they had not acknowledged noncompliance but were willingly agreeing to consultation, the use of the consultants should be outside of the purview of the suit and should be done solely on a voluntary basis.

---

9. R.A.J. v. Miller, R.A.J. Review Panel Tenth Report to the Court, July 1987, p. 71.

148   State Hospital Reform: Why Was It So Hard to Accomplish?

Disagreement over this issue was intense until it became apparent that such disagreement would cause the Defendants to refuse to use the consultants. The Parties therefore agreed that the consultants would review the presence of psychosocial programming in six of the eight state hospitals.[10] Specifically, the consultants would make recommendations concerning training and consultation that they would provide in a second phase of this project. The Parties agreed that the consultants would submit a report and the Defendants would create a corrective action plan aimed at dealing with the issues that they chose to address based upon the consultants' recommendations. The Monitor selected Dr. Robert Liberman and his colleagues as the consultants.[11] [12] Site visits were conducted by Psychiatric Rehabilitation Consultants (PRC), Dr. Liberman's consulting group during the summer of 1988. In November of 1988 Psychiatric Rehabilitation Consultants conducted a four-day workshop of findings of the assessments, their recommendations, and concepts of psychosocial rehabilitation. This workshop was attended by hospital superintendents, medical directors, and key program staff. The consultants then revised their report and submitted a final report in January of 1989.[13]

The Monitor decided to present an abstract of the findings of the consultants in his Thirteenth Report to the Court because he believed the findings substantiated previous findings of the Review Panel and their consultants. Generally the consultants found the following positive conditions in the hospitals:

- The multiple disability units for the mentally ill and mentally retarded and transitional living units for the general psychi-

---

10. R.A.J. v. Jones, Stipulated Agreement on the Use of Psychiatric Rehabilitation Consultants, July 1988.

11. Liberman, R.P., Jacobs, H.E., Boone, S., Falloon, I.R.H., Blackwell, G., and Wallace, C.J., "New Methods for Rehabilitating Chronic Mental Patients," in J.A. Talbott (ed.), *Psychiatric Disability: Clinical, Administrative, and Legal Aspects*. Washington, DC: American Psychiatric Press.

12. Liberman, R.P., and Associates, Psychiatric Rehabilitation of Chronic Mental Patients. Washington, DC: American Psychiatric Press, 1987.

13. Psychiatric Rehabilitation Consultants, *Needs Assessment for Psychiatric Rehabilitation in the Texas State Hospitals*, submitted to the R.A.J. Court Monitor, January 1989.

atric population demonstrated excellent psychosocial treating procedures and techniques. These programs often contained well-structured curriculum, and leaders and trainers who were prepared for their sessions; activities that were delivered in groups of manageable size; and program leaders who reviewed and adjusted the training programs to meet the needs of the patients.

- Several of these programs were using formal functional assessment tools to determine the patient's functional needs.

- Most of the hospitals had good to excellent facilities to conduct psychosocial rehabilitation.

- Initial psychiatric and social assessments were often well done but the findings of the assessments were not always integrated in a useful way into an individualized treatment plan.

- Psychotropic medications were usually within acceptable ranges or exceptions to the usual use were adequately documented.

- There was evidence of regular reviews for tardive dyskinesia documented in the patients' records.[14]

The psychiatric rehabilitation consultants presented recommendations aimed at addressing problems. These included:

- Treatment plans and goals should be more specific, better prioritized, and relevant to the reason for the patient's admission to the hospital.

- Functional assessments on the acute, intermediate, and extended units (general psychiatric units) needed improvement.

- Treatment plans needed more specific goals with criteria to include operational statements of changes in patient's functional status and behavior rather than focusing on measures of patient's attendance and participation in service.

- Treatment objectives needed to be written in measurable terms.

---

14. R.A.J. v. Jones, The Court Monitor's Thirteenth Report to the Court, February 1989.

- There should be better concordance between written treatment plans and the actual services delivered.

- There should be more uniform implementation of educational and behavior therapy programs across the units.

- Many unmotivated patients were inactive in day halls during program periods. Programs appeared to be underutilized.

- Activity groups should be increased from three to four to six to eight patients each and people should be encouraged to attend.

- Patients unable to leave the unit should have appropriate psychosocial programming suited to their needs provided on the units. This should include training in self-care skills, training in anger management, and training in basic conversational skills.

- Physicians' progress notes need better justification for initial and maintenance psychopharmacology as well as for changing drugs or drug doses.

- The rationale for psychotropic medication should be more specific and should include desired changes in target symptoms.

- Discharge criteria should be formulated in terms of "controlling and managing symptoms" and the attainment of functional skills useful for community living rather than "absence" of symptoms or signs of mental disorder.

- Goals should be formulated in positive terms rather than negative terms.

- Treatment should focus upon the reduction of negative symptoms. Negative symptoms such as withdrawal, apathy, disorganization, poor social relationships, and lack of functioning skills are not highly responsive to psychotropic medications. Skill training and other behavioral rehabilitation methods should address these negative symptoms.[15]

When the PRC report was presented to TXMHMR, the Defendants adamantly stated that the action plan was outside the Settlement Agreement and that this was a voluntary effort at improving

---

15. Ibid.

conditions in the hospitals. This position previously had been reluctantly accepted by the Plaintiffs and Monitor and was represented in the Stipulated Agreement.[16] An action plan was presented by TXMHMR but an overall systems approach for the implementation of psychosocial programming at the hospitals was never implemented. Each hospital developed its own implementation plan. Four hospitals fully developed psychosocial rehabilitation programming and contracted independently with Dr. Liebermann's consultants. The other hospitals were less focused in their development of programs and did not use outside consultation. Each hospital did commit to developing an extended care unit with psychosocial programming

The Plaintiffs and Monitor accepted the Defendants' position that the development of these programs was outside the purview of the Settlement Agreement. Compliance, therefore, could not be based upon whether a psychosocial program was developed but rather would need to be based upon whether individualized treatment was being provided to patients. The development of psychosocial programming, which began in 1989, went on for several years. Several hospitals have maintained complex programs. This exploration into psychosocial rehabilitation, however, did not greatly clarify questions about how individualized treatment is recognized and measured.

By the time the Monitor and his consultants were collecting data for the Fourteenth Report to the Court they had accepted the fact that the development of psychosocial programs would not be used as a measure of individualized treatment. They returned their attention to the revision of the clinical instrument. The revisions of this case reading monitoring form all examined the presence of assessments, case formulation, a treatment plan, the provision of services, the monitoring of the effects of service, and the reformulation of the case.

As the Monitor and the consultants continued talking about the problems of individualizing care they focused more and more upon the issue of case formulation as a primary component to service delivery. The consultants observed that in those cases where there ap-

---

16. R.A.J. v. Jones, Stipulated Agreement on the use of Psychiatric Rehabilitation Consultants, July 1988.

peared to be good individualized treatment, significant clinical leadership was apparent. The psychiatrist, psychologist, or sometimes a social worker, often played the organizing function of formulating the case.

When that function was not performed well, individualized treatment occurred less frequently. The consultants began recognizing both the presence and absence of clinical thinking which they decided was a clinical formulation.

After reviewing hundreds of diagnostic assessments and treatment plans, it was apparent that staff recording contained some consistent characteristics. The nature of note taking was quite uniform regardless of whether notes were provided by paraprofessional staff such as mental health workers or professional staff such as psychologists or psychiatrists. Specifically the notes tended to be like those one would expect from descriptions of a naive observer. This appeared to reflect a misunderstood notion of being "objective." It was impossible to see any inferential thinking by clinicians. In addition, the wording of treatment plans tended to be very fixed and repetitive, show little individualized understanding of the patient. There was a tendency to give formulaic descriptions of problems and packaged interventions.

It became increasingly clear that there was an absence of any hypothesized conceptualization to explain the individual illness of a given patient as it related to that patient's life and circumstances. The logical place for such a statement appeared to be in an area marked "Formulation or Case Summary" on the treatment plan document. This classification appeared to be taken as a requirement to summarize the facts of the case rather than as a statement of clinical thinking.

As the Court Monitor's consultants attempted to understand how and why there were problems in the area of case formulation they had to define formulation for themselves. They decided that a psychiatric formulation is the synthesis of a patient's biographic history with psychiatric knowledge and theory to produce an explanation for why the patient's condition is what it is. The formulation is based upon the information contained in the biological, psychological, social, familial, and psychosocial assessments and evaluations. The formulation is a set of hypotheses about how and why the patient got to be where he or she currently is. These hypotheses are based upon the most relevant factors in the patient's situation. The formulation

Measurement of Psychiatric Care 153

process of raising hypotheses therefore sets the cornerstone for further treatment by defining treatment issues and priorities. The formulation makes explicit the logic behind the treatment plan because it demonstrates the clinician's thinking about why things have happened and what needs to be addressed to change the current conditions.

Sperry, Gudeman, Blackwell, and Faulkner published a useful synthesis of different schools of psychiatric formulation which states that a good formulation contains descriptive, explanatory, and treatment-prognostic components.[17] The descriptive component tells what happened. The explanatory component answers why it happened and the treatment-prognostic component presents a plan or working hypothesis about what can be done about it and what is the likelihood of success.[18]

The term formulation evokes the memory of the concept of psychodynamic formulation. This is a narrow definition of the concept of formulation. In a broader sense, formulation takes a comprehensive picture of the patient's functioning. It includes the consideration of biological, psychological, social, and familial factors. The priority setting among these factors is based upon the client condition. The client's condition indicates what psychiatric knowledge and theory should be utilized. In this manner the formulation truly individualizes treatment planning. If the client's condition is primarily caused by an organic impairment, the primary focus will be upon managing the biological condition. Attention may be paid to the effects of the condition upon the client's social and family interactions. Another patient may present problems that are a clear mix of biological, psychological, and family issues. The formulation is a telling of the patient's story in such a way that the causes are made clear and the interrelationships between biological, psychological, social, and familial factors are also made explicit.

A case formulation is very different from a summary of a patient's history. A formulation is a statement of clinical thinking. It therefore

---

17. Sperry, L., Gudeman, J.E., Blackwell, B., and Faulkner, L.R., *Psychiatric Case Formulations*, American Psychiatric Press, Inc., Washington, DC, 1992.
18. Ibid.

reflects something about the treating clinician. A summary is a condensed description of the case; it can stand alone. A person could read a summary and have a capsule view of what has happened to a patient. A formulation does not stand alone. It implies a knowledge of the historical and other descriptive materials of the case. The formulation does not have to repeat this information.

A formulation needs to address the question of why the hospitalization has occurred at a certain time. This requires some attention to precipitance. A frequent pattern in describing readmission of a chronically ill patient is to describe the episodes simply as one more reoccurrence of an ongoing illness or simply to relate it to the failure to take medication. Other important precipitating events are often ignored even though they are mentioned as a part of the phase of descriptive information gathering.

As the clinician thinks diagnostically he or she can choose from among a wide range of theoretical frameworks using those that are most relevant to a particular patient. All possible bases or positions need not be covered. Part of the clinician's thinking is the choice of a useful framework for a specific case. A point central to formulation is the understanding that it represents a hypothesis and as such requires testing. Testing comes in the form of treatments. If a hypothesis is correct, one should be able to predict that certain treatments will be effective in certain ways within a certain time frame. The failure of this to occur as predicted should lead to a reconsideration of the formulation.

A good formulation should help determine the priority of treatment interventions. Certain treatment needs may be unaddressable until others are dealt with. For instance, a highly psychotic patient may have treatment needs that can not be addressed until the psychosis is at least partially treated.

Furthermore, a good formulation will indicate when certain problems or symptoms are secondary to others. A good example of this is the patient who shows impairment in basic self-care when psychotic but quite able to handle these matters when the psychosis is under control. In such a case it is inappropriate to spend hours of time training basic skills such as grooming and hygiene when these will improve automatically when the patient's psychosis is treated. A good understanding of the mechanisms of treatment will prevent this kind of mindless treatment planning.

A good formulation will allow the clinician to choose between several approaches to the same problem, selecting the one most likely to be helpful given the mechanism of the patient's difficulty. An example of this is the patient who is noncompliant with medication who is assigned to medication education sessions in a rather automatic manner regardless of the reason for his or her noncompliance. In truth, education is only helpful for those patients who fail to comply because they do not understand basic matters about the medication. Many patients fail to comply because of other reasons such as the subtle side effects of their medication, their own denial of illness, or loss of self-esteem that they associate with needing medication. In such cases other treatment interventions addressing these issues will be required.

A formulation allows a treatment plan to make a rational use of "stock treatments." Most facilities have a range of available group classes that address common problems. These have not been designed with specific individual patients in mind. The use of such "stock treatments" is acceptable as long as careful thought is given to how and why an individual patient will benefit from the treatment. A good formulation can provide the logic for why a particular group intervention is relevant to a given patient.

A critical point is that the formulation needs to allow the clinician to get beyond a knee-jerk matching of the symptoms with an intervention. This can be illustrated well by a discussion of the issue of aggression. Aggression is a common problem in the state hospitals. There is a tendency to apply certain interventions automatically to all aggressive patients, yet the truth is there are many reasons for aggression. Aggression that results from delusional paranoid thinking may best be treated with antipsychotic medication. Other acts of aggression are the results of low frustration tolerance, lack of skills in negotiation and problem solving, or issues of secondary gain. Each form of aggression has its own mechanism and hence its own relevant treatment.

The Monitor and his consultants focused upon formulation as a critical key to the provision of good clinical care in a state hospital. In essence, they formulated that the lack of clear, explicit clinical thinking through a formulation contributed to inadequate treatment planning and the lack of individualized treatment. At one point while the Defendants and Monitor were still arguing about clinical care, some TXMHMR staff stated that the consultants were obsessing about formulation. The value of the formulation process as a key to the provision of good clinical care seems to have been borne out through the improvement of care caused by the five years of implementation of the QSO process. This process will be explained in greater detail in Dr. Axelrad's chapter on the QSO clinical instruments which will illustrate how treatment was assessed in the Texas hospitals from 1992 through 1997 when the case was dismissed from the jurisdiction of the Court. Formulation was only one of twenty-one issues measured through the QSO instrument on individualized treatment. However, it was the issue that during the early implementation phase was consistently most often missed. The fact that this item was the item scored most negatively made it important for both the R.A.J. consultants and the QSO consultants to define formulation, agree among themselves what the components of a formulation were, and actively consult with the hospitals on how to do formulations. The QSO consultants became as convinced that formulation was a key to making care understandable and explicit as the R.A.J. consultants were.

This chapter relates a meandering journey where psychiatric consultants for the Review Panel and Court Monitor attempted to conceptualize why the treatment in the Texas state hospitals appeared to be clinically inadequate. Much of the journey was conducted through a hostile environment. This was because the Monitor and the consultants were criticizing treatment in the hospitals, saying that it was inadequate, and then attempting to diagnose how and why it was inadequate. The Defendants did not accept the allegations of inadequacy and stated that the consultants were making biased, subjective statements. The Defendants had not asked for the criticism and were not happy that they were in a place legally where they had outside critics in a position to make such judgments. This situation became more and more adversarial and acrimonious.

During the ten most adversarial years, from 1982–1992, the Panel and then the Monitor's focus moved from looking at the psychiatric treatment process to looking at the type of psychiatric programming apparently most appropriate for the chronically mentally ill, i.e, psychosocial programming, to refocusing on the psychiatric treatment process.

The Defendant's use of the Romeo v. Youngberg standard of professional judgment may have complicated the search for an understanding of what were the causes for the problems of individualized treatment in the state hospitals. This standard implied that any professional judgment was as good as any other professional judgment. This position was an apparently adequate legal defense against the criticism of clinical practices. However, this defense interfered with the examination of problems with clinical care. Because of this defense there was no incentive for the Defendants to work with the Monitor to really understand the level of clinical competence in the hospitals.

It was only after the negotiation of the QSO process and then the negotiations that the consultants for the both the Monitor's team and the QSO team had to go through to make operational the items contained in the clinical questionnaire, that clinicians representing the Monitor and the state hospital system were able to recognize that they did share values, a knowledge base, and the clinical thinking needed to define definitions of clinical practice. These clinicians were able to come to agreement about the adequacy of the assessments, the formulations, the treatment plan, treatment provision, and reformulation on a case by case basis. They were able to articulate what they were looking for in terms of the elements of care and gradually staffs in the hospitals began to demonstrate their clinical thinking more clearly in the records in a manner that met the standards defined through the clinical instruments. This was a long process. It took five years and over ten site visit reviews to the hospitals during that time frame.

It was only after the adversarial atmosphere of the lawsuit was diminished appreciably through the negotiation of the QSO process and the development of the monitoring instruments that consultants for the Defendants and the clinical staffs at the hospitals were really capable of cooperating with the Monitor and his clinical consultants to consider how conditions could be improved.

Chapter 8

The Excursion into the Community

David Pharis

Once the parties to the lawsuit, the legislature, the media, and other observers of the suit became aware that compliance with the many requirements had become a protracted struggle, many critics of the suit charged that the lawsuit was a bottomless pit and that, in fact, compliance was a moving target. The most vocal critics were administrators of the Texas Department of Mental Health and Mental Retardation and several members of the legislature. They perceived that the Review Panel kept creating issues and that once one issue was resolved the Panel brought up other issues. They also maintained that the Plaintiffs' attorneys actively participated in this process. The critics' opposition to the Court's involvement and their concerns that the Panel was creating issues was most intense concerning the issues of community aftercare. The attorneys for the Defendants took the position that there was no constitutional requirement that the state provide adequate community aftercare. The Defendants argued this position forcefully throughout the life of the lawsuit and in fact intensified this argument during the final years of this suit.

However, the initial involvement in community aftercare was entered by the Defendants willingly through the issue's inclusion in the 1981 Settlement Agreement. In this document, the Defendants agreed to take appropriate action to provide patients released from their hospitals with the proper transition and follow-up care from the hospital setting to the nonhospital setting. Each client was to have appropriate discharge planning and continuity of care. Continuity of care was to be assured across regions and each community mental health center was to provide such services.[1] In the 1980's the Defendants had an adequate continuity of care rule which defined the process by which a referral was to be made from the state hospital to the mental health center for follow-up.[2]

---

1. R.A.J. v. Miller, Settlement Agreement, April 1981.
2. State of Texas, *Texas Administrative Code*, Chapter 534, 1982.

159

The Defendants' initial action plan for initiating the 1981 Settlement Agreement carried action steps by which the continuity of care rule was to be implemented.[3] This action plan contained the usual provisions of having hospital admissions prescreened by community center personnel to establish the appropriateness of the use of the state hospital and have center personnel involved with the treatment team through the processes of treatment to discharge. This initial action plan included the steps for adequate budget requests for this activity for the next legislative session. The policy for adequate community aftercare therefore existed in 1982 although there were many reports that screening and referrals between the hospitals and the community centers were not taking place.

The Court became more involved in community aftercare issues after the Court found the Defendants out of compliance with major requirements of the case.[4]

After the Court ordered the implementation of the staffing ratios by August 1985, the Defendants asked the Court to accept the concept that compliance with the staffing ratios could be met through either the hiring of additional staff in the hospitals or through the reduction of the patient populations in each hospital. The Court accepted this concept under the requirement that patients discharged from the facilities to the community would be discharged to "adequately staffed facilities sufficient to provide appropriate treatment."[5]

An unanticipated side effect of the implementation of the staffing requirements was the development of a mechanism of putting money into the community called the $35.50 Program. The Texas legislature in a special session in 1985 appropriated approximately $17 million to fund the staffing requirements. When the Defendants requested the alternative of complying with the staff requirements through the reduction of the population in the hospitals, the Commissioner conceived of a means of transferring the monies which would have been used for the hiring of staff to community programs. The number of

---

3. Texas Department of Mental Health and Mental Retardation, "Defendants' Action Plan," filed with Court January 1994.

4. R.A.J. v. Miller, Memorandum Opinion and Order, April 1984.

5. R.A.J. v. Miller, Order from Hearing on Stipulated Recommendation of Remedies, June 1984.

people that each mental health authority (MHA) had in a state hospital was calculated for a particular baseline period of time. The MHA's then were notified that for every day that they reduced below the baseline utilization rate they could earn $35.50 per day. For example, if an MHA had been averaging 100 people in state hospitals and reduced that average to 85 people they would earn (15 x $35 x the number of the days of the reduction). The earnings would be calculated on a quarterly basis and the payment of funds, therefore, were based on the bed-day reduction of the previous quarter.

The $35.50 Program created an incentive for the mental health authorities to focus on serving the chronically mentally ill in the community. The emphasis on a reduction of hospital bed days and the need to maintain a reduction once funds had been earned and services had been financed were direct results of this program. The $35.50 Program provided approximately $38 million of new money into the community mental health system from the summer of 1985 through the summer of 1988.

The decision to attempt to meet the staffing ratios requirements through the reduction of the populations of the hospitals during the late months of 1984 caused a high degree of public concern that TXMHMR was inappropriately dumping clients from the state hospitals to inadequate community resources. This public concern was caused by adverse publicity about one hospital's attempt to reduce the length of stay of patients in key programs through the aggressive use of psychotropic medications and through the negative publicity generated by patients being placed on buses from Austin to Houston with an overnight placement at a local shelter. Aftercare planning in this situation consisted of a bus ticket and a one-night stay at the Salvation Army. The appropriate question was, does this constitute a referral to an adequately staffed facility sufficient to provide appropriate treatment?

An evidentiary hearing to examine the appropriateness of the Defendants' efforts at reducing the hospitals' population was held in March 1985. The executive directors of the community mental health centers in Houston, Dallas, San Antonio, El Paso, Austin, and Beaumont were invited by the Court to testify regarding discharge planning and the availability of services in their area.

The Review Panel examined a 10 percent sample of patients discharged from the eight state hospitals during the period from June 1,

1984, to November 30, 1984 (583 cases). The purpose of this analysis was to determine the presence of an aftercare plan and follow-up appointments in patient records. The Panel determined that 118 clients in its sample of 583 (21%) did not have an aftercare plan and an additional 77 plans (13%) were "of the most minimal nature." There were explanations for the lack of a plan in all records that did not have plans except for 43 clients (7%).

The Defendants argued that there was an explanation for the lack of aftercare plans for all but 43 clients (7% of the sample). These explanations were discharge against medical advice, discharge by the Court, discharge from unauthorized discharge status (runaways), client refused aftercare plan, and the client left the state. The Defendants argued in the Court that such actions absolved them of responsibility for further case planning. The Defendants argued that this 21 percent of the sample has effectively removed itself from the Defendants' responsibility for service provision. No aftercare appointment was listed in the records of 190 clients (33%); 5 percent of the sample had no explanation for the lack of an appointment while 86 clients (15%) lacked both a plan and an appointment for aftercare services. There were explanations documented for all but 11 clients. Again the explanations, included discharge from unauthorized discharge, discharge against medical advice, discharged by the Courts and refused aftercare plan.

The average length of time between discharge and the first follow-up appointment at a community center for those patients who had appointments was 13 days. There was evidence that there was a referral phone call between the hospital and the aftercare agency 76 percent of the time.[6]

Several of the community mental center directors testified that they were unable to provide adequate services to patients discharged to them from the state hospitals. Most of the directors categorized the services for such patients as "minimally adequate."

The Court concluded that many clients discharged from the hospitals were receiving services which were minimally adequate and that

---

6. R.A.J. v. Miller, R.A.J. Review Panel Special Report to the Court No. III, March 1985.

minimally adequate services did not comply with the court order that community alternatives must be "adequately staffed facilities sufficient to provide appropriate treatment."[7]

A legislative response to the Court's 1984 finding of noncompliance was the formation of the Legislative Oversight Committee on Mental Health and Mental Retardation which filed a report in February 1985.[8] This committee recommended the development of the definition of priority service population for the Department of Mental Health and Mental Retardation and the definition of core services available to this population. These services included 24-hour emergency screening, rapid stabilization services, crisis hospitalization, initial assessment performed in the community, medication services, and case management services. These services were mandated by the Texas senate in SB 633 in 1985 but unfortunately the funds for the development for these services were not appropriated.

During 1986 the parties and the Review Panel negotiated criteria for adequate community aftercare. The five criteria for community based aftercare were as follows:

1. The mental health authority must make a good faith effort to make available and accessible those services specified in the community aftercare plans for patients discharged to their care for as long as the mental health authority determined that the client needs these services.

2. The mental health authority will make follow-up appointments for all persons referred for aftercare services and will document efforts made to assist the client in keeping the appointment.

3. The mental health authority will document outreach efforts made specifically in the effort to extend services specified in the community aftercare plan for hard-to-reach clients.

4. The mental health authority will make a good faith effort to make available case management services to those clients who qualify according to TXMHMR criteria.

---

7. R.A.J. v. Miller, Findings of Fact and Conclusion of Law, June 1985.

8. Texas Legislative Oversight Committee on Mental Health and Mental Retardation, "Report to the Texas Legislature," February 1985.

5. The mental health authority will make a good faith effort to arrange for nonclinical support for patients in cases in which the Department assessment indicates that long-term hospitalization and chronicity of mental illness justifies such action. This provision will apply only in those situations in which no other resources are available.[9]

The Court adopted these criteria as the means for measuring further questions about the adequacy of community care.

Howard Goldman, M.D., Ph.D., from the University of Maryland developed methodology to measure the five criteria for the efficacy of community aftercare. His first study of the adequacy of community aftercare, completed in 1988, concluded that 56 percent of the records that he reviewed met the requirements for compliance, 28 percent partially met compliance, and 15 percent did not meet compliance with the requirements of the five criteria for aftercare.[10] Defendants disagreed with the method of the study, although they considered the findings to represent substantial compliance. The Plaintiffs considered the results to represent noncompliance. The results of this study were considered inconclusive by the Court and the Court ordered that the aftercare issue be further evaluated.

Dr. Goldman conducted a second adequacy of community aftercare evaluation in 1990.[11] Defendants insisted on negotiating the technical design of this study. The Plaintiffs' attorney, the Defendants, the Court Monitor, and Dr. Goldman were involved in several long adversarial meetings. Defendants again insisted upon defining the study population as not containing people they considered had withdrawn from their service authority. They also insisted upon the inclusion of the concept of good faith effort before each requirement. The study design, produced through the adversarial negotiation process, was based upon the premise that the provision of aftercare services should only be measured for those people who made themselves available for such services. The reason that this premise was accepted by the Plaintiffs and the Panel was that the Defendants

---

9. R.A.J. v. Miller, Recommendation 35, October 1986.

10. R.A.J. v. Miller; Goldman, H., "Report on the Adequacy of Community Aftercare Services," March 1988.

11. R.A.J. v. Miller; Goldman, H., "Report on Results of an Evaluation of Compliance with Aftercare Criteria in Texas," November 1990.

made it clear that their willing participation in this study was contingent upon acceptance of this premise.

The overall universe of people discharged from the hospitals was reduced therefore by the number of people who left the hospital against medical advice, refused ongoing services, went to jail rather than mental health facilities, or left the area without a request for a mental health referral. This deletion of hard-to-reach clients reduced the sample by approximately 20 percent.

This study identified that 80 percent of the patients discharged from the state hospitals were receiving the aftercare services as they were defined by the five criteria. The finding that 80 percent of the reduced population received services may not be surprising or questionable. Eighty percent of those people who make themselves available for services actually received services. The concern here could be that an additional 20 percent of a very vulnerable population did not receive services because they made themselves unavailable. This group conceivably would be the most needful of the mentally ill. A more complete examination of the Goldman studies is made in Chapter 9.

One should note that the findings from the first study conducted by the Review Panel in 1985 are similar to Dr. Goldman's findings in 1990. In both studies approximately 20 percent of the population discharged from the hospitals made themselves unavailable for aftercare services. Regardless of whether a mental health agency has responsibility for providing service to this population it can be argued that many clients who drop out of the service system are those with great need for mental health services. Many clients, family members, and advocates for the mentally ill consistently complained to the Review Panel and Court Monitor about the inadequacy of community services. These complaints often stated that clients were discharged inappropriately from the state hospitals before their mental illness was in remission and that they often did not have adequate follow-up supportive plans. There were often allegations that clients did not have adequate places to live, income, or support services as needed. These allegations were in conflict with the findings of the Goldman reports. The allegations therefore reflected firmly held subjective beliefs in conflict with more objective evaluation.

One reason that administrators and the legislature complained about the Panel or the Monitor creating new issues was that as the Panel or the Monitor investigated complaints they raised the question of whether the incident represented compliance with the requirements of the Settlement Agreement. In terms of aftercare the question became, does this represent referral to facilities staffed adequately to meet treatment needs and did the situation meet the requirements of the five criteria?

The Whisper Oaks complaint, the Devine complaint, and the Hospitality House complaint led to three investigations which brought some interesting insights into the nature of aftercare provision in the state. The Review Panel investigated the effects of a limited budget upon a contract with the Whisper Oaks Personal Care Home in 1987 when the Plaintiffs' attorney asked the Panel to examine the situation where clients were having to leave the home due to inadequate funds from TXMHMR to fund them through their contract period.[12] The contract between the personal care home and the state hospital was aimed at taking care of people discharged from the hospital or preventing people from being hospitalized by the provision of the less restrictive residential care. The contract was supported by the $35.50 Program. At the time of the crisis some twenty people were in the personal care home when it was determined that the budget was being overspent and that for the rest of the year only thirteen people could be supported by the remaining funds. Seven people, therefore, were discharged from the facility. The Plaintiffs' attorney asked the Review Panel to determine whether these discharges were decided upon clinical need or upon the financial crisis.

The Review Panel concluded that compromised clinical decision making had unquestionably occurred when the hospital administrators realized that they had been overspending $35.50 monies and therefore had to reduce spending. Although several of the patients who left the personal care home were considered short term residents, there was no indication in the records that they would normally have been leaving at the time they left. They left when they did due to the financial crisis. Clinical decisions were therefore determined by this financial situation. The outreach department of the hospital did make a clear effort to minimize any possible harm to clients as they left the facility by providing follow-up services. At the same time, however, the clients lost the structured living situation which they had appeared to be needing and using appropriately.

12. R.A.J. v. Miller, Special Report to the Court: The Whisper Oaks Licensed Personal Care Home, March 1987.

The Review Panel maintained that the situation raised disturbing questions about building a program on soft money which might not be available to adequately support the program in the long run.[13] The Defendants disagreed with the Panel's conclusion that compromised clinical decision making occurred. The tone of the Defendants' comments revealed some increasing frustration on the Defendants' part about the activities of the Panel.

> The Department's $35.50 program is an innovative funding mechanism to discourage inappropriate admissions to the state hospitals and encourage the growth of community-based alternatives. Contrary to the Panel's assertions, the issue highlighted by the Whisper Oaks situation is not that the $35.50 program rests on soft money but that the need for services exceeds the resources of the Department. This is, however, not news. And the Department should not be faulted for attempting to provide quality services just because they are incapable of providing the quantity of services required to meet the needs of all mentally ill persons....

> Although the Rusk State hospital and the Texas Department of Mental Health and Mental Retardation appreciate the expression of opinion by the Review Panel, the hospital and the Department respectfully disagree with the Panel's conclusion that "compromised clinical decision making occurred...." The Panel apparently believes that such compromised decisions occurred with regard to two residents of the facility. The decisions made in this matter were made by persons whose expertise lies in the area of case management and other types of community based services. Those persons worked with the residents of the Whisper Oaks facility on an ongoing basis and had personal knowledge of their illnesses, abilities, strengths, and weaknesses that could not be gained by the Review Panel members or Plaintiffs' attorney during visits to the facility or through review of records. This type of decision making was, and continues to be, part of the staff's professional responsibility; and while the opinions of periodic visitors are welcome, the hospital and the Department cannot allow those

---

13. Ibid.

opinions to be substituted for the professional judgment of its outreach staff, who are truly experts in this area of mental health services.[14]

The question of whether patients were losing services due to lack of financial resources was never resolved by the Court but the situation was discussed in the media and it did illustrate how clinical thinking can be influenced by financial reality.

During the fall of 1989 the R.A.J. Court Monitor received reports about the placement of a large number of clients from the San Antonio State Hospital to a number of board and care homes in Devine, Texas, and the surrounding area of Medina County. Many of these homes were operated by members of a large extended family. The informants suggested that these facilities might not be adequate to meet the service needs of the clients and that there might be problems with the lack of mental health aftercare services. They suggested that no one was taking responsibility for the placement of theses patients or was coordinating their follow-up care and posed the question of whether this type of discharge to board and care facilities was what was anticipated in the Judge's Order concerning referral to adequately staffed facilities to meet the treatment needs of clients.

It appeared that during the previous ten years that San Antonio State Hospital, which at that time was the mental health authority for the county, had placed up to 300 patients from the state hospital to these facilities. Other patients have been discharged to theses facilities from the Rio Grande Center and more recently from Kerrville State Hospital. During the time that San Antonio State Hospital was making its numerous discharges, that state hospital's outreach department was responsible for the psychiatric care for that area.

In 1987, however, the boundaries of the mental health authority were altered and Kerrville State Hospital became responsible for this area. The Kerrville State Hospital outreach department therefore had been providing mental health services to some of these clients. Devine, Texas, is approximately thirty miles from San Antonio and ninety miles from Kerrville.

San Antonio State Hospital had discharged 274 clients from their facility to the board and care homes from 1981 through 1987. In

---

14. R.A.J. v. Miller, "Defendant's Comments on R.A.J. Review Panel Report on Whisper Oaks Licensed Personal Care Home," April 1987.

The Excursion into the Community   169

1987 Kerrville State Hospital picked up this area as part of their outreach department jurisdiction. Kerrville State Hospital received the transfer of these 274 clients as closed cases from the San Antonio State Hospital Outreach Department. Kerrville State Hospital apparently did not open the cases or investigate whether these people might need psychiatric services. After taking Medina County as a service area, Kerrville State Hospital Outreach Department opened 94 cases from these homes. There were no duplications among the 274 closed cases from San Antonio State Hospital and the 94 open cases of the Kerrville State Hospital Outreach Department were not a duplicate list of clients; they were all different people.

In December 1989 the Court Monitor and two psychiatric consultants, the Deputy Commissioner of Mental Health Services for the Texas Department of Mental Health and Mental Retardation, the Superintendent of Kerrville State Hospital, and five Kerrville State Hospital Outreach Department staff toured five board and care homes, three personal care homes, and a 48-bed custodial care facility. While touring the facilities they looked at the physical environment, observed patients, asked the operators questions about care provided by the homes and about how the patients received psychiatric and medical care.[15]

The board and care homes and the personal care homes provided very basic room and board. The facilities ranged from clean but extremely stark to clean with some attempt to provide a homelike environment through the use of pleasant inexpensive furniture and decorations.

Texas law required that mental health authorities develop minimal standards for board and care homes. The mental health authority could only place clients in homes that meet the standards. Compliance with the standards was voluntary and board and care homes could operate outside of these standards as long as they got referrals from other sources than the mental health authority. Personal care homes were licensed by the Texas Department of Health.

The funding for these board and care homes was basically from the patients' social security disability checks. The patients received

---

15. R.A.J. v. Jones, "The Court Monitor's Report on Board and Care Homes in Devine, Texas," January 1990.

$365 per month for their social security disability. The owners of the board and care homes took that check, cashed it and gave the patient $25 in cash for their personal needs. The remainder was used by the owner of the board and care as their fee for board and care. This averaged to about $10 per day per person. Out of this the board and care provider was to feed, cloth, house the boarder, and make a living for his family, i.e., realize a profit. In the personal care home the provider received $9.00 per day for support of the client in addition to the SSI disability payment. This additional payment came from the Texas Department of Health. The rationale for this difference in cost was that clients in personal care homes were more disabled than those in board and care homes and needed more personalized services including help in feeding, dressing, and the supervised administration of medication.

The providers, however, said that the clients in the personal care homes were no different from those in the board and care homes and that the provider in reality provided the same kind of services to clients in each of the different types of homes.

There were two systems of care for the provision of medical and psychiatric services for the clients in these board and care and personal care homes. Theses two systems appeared to function separately from each other with little or no formal coordination. Several community doctors served this population and at the same time a portion of the population was served by the Kerrville State Hospital Outreach Department. That department, however, did not consider all of the clients who had been discharged from the state hospital to these facilities to be on their active case load. An internist from San Antonio brought a nurse and medical technician one day per week to the Medina County area and went through the board and care homes. The clients in each board and care home were therefore monitored by this internist approximately once per month. He handled both medical and psychiatric situations and prescribed psychotropic medications. All of the board and care and personal care providers worked closely with this physician. The providers felt that they could call him in an emergency and that he would either deal with the situation during his next visit or refer for emergency hospital care to a psychiatrist in San Antonio who would hospitalize these patients in a private hospital and receive Medicaid payments for their inpatient psychiatric treatment. Once a patient was discharged from the psychiatric hospital he or she usually returned back to the board and care home and to the internist's care.

The Kerrville State Hospital Outreach Department had approximately 100 clients from the area on their active case load. About 45 of those were picked up at the time of the transfer and the remainder had become active cases after that. These people were also seen by the internist and some of them might have been hospitalized by the San Antonio psychiatrist.

One board and care and personal care provider had a very good working relationship with the Kerrville State Hospital Outreach Department and most of the clients at this facility were on the caseload there. Other providers, however, had a less close working relationship with the Kerrville State Hospital Outreach Department. Several providers told us that they preferred the San Antonio community doctors because they had dealt with them for a long time and had a greater sense of trust that the doctors would be responsive to their statements that the patients were becoming disturbed. They also believed that it was easier to hospitalize the patients in the San Antonio community hospitals than at Kerrville State Hospital.

A physician from the Kerrville State Hospital Outreach Department expressed concern to the Monitor about these coordination problems between the outreach department and the community doctors. He stated that there had been times when these community physicians had changed his medications on a patient without communication or coordination with him.

There appeared to be a major unanswered question about who was providing psychiatric care to these clients and who had authority over the case. One question was whether the Kerrville State Hospital Outreach Department should have psychiatric aftercare responsibility for all clients discharged from the state hospital. Another question was if and when a patient had two physicians, who was primarily responsible for the psychiatric treatment? Questions also rose concerning whether the doctors worked for the patients or the homes. Most of these patients did not have guardians and therefore should be considered in charge of their own affairs. The impaired patients in these facilities did not appear to be in control of decision making around these questions. It appeared however that decisions about treatment were being made by the board and care providers rather than the patients.

There was no evidence of organized programming at any of these facilities. The only forms of recreation observed were individual people walking around the grounds of a facility, one staff and younger resident playing bingo with two older residents, a group of men and women sitting in the living room of the homes watching television, and eight to ten men standing along the walls of a barren plywood shed smoking.

The Kerrville State Hospital Outreach Department provided some day activities at a centralized psychosocial workshop. They picked clients up and took them to these activities. The board and care providers conducted occasional trips to town for shopping and movies.

Most of these facilities were actually not in the town of Devine but rather were in the county in isolated rural areas. Many of the providers of these facilities were members of a large extended family and several different facilities were actually next to each other. They however were all on rural roads and clients were quite isolated from town. Clients were kept in fenced yards and were not permitted to leave the facilities on their own.

The Court Monitor's report raised questions about whether the placement of clients in facilities such as these board and care homes met the Court's expectation that clients are placed in adequately staffed facilities to meet treatment needs. In a second report the Monitor questioned whether these clients were receiving the individualized treatment required by the five community aftercare criteria.[16] Negotiations with the Parties after the filing of these two reports resulted in an action plan Kerrville State Hospital's Outreach Department agreed to do assessments of all clients in these facilities and offer follow-up care. Although the jurisdictional issues between the physicians were discussed, these went largely unaddressed or resolved in the action plan.[17]

During the summer and winter of 1985 TXMHMR proposed to the Review Panel that the Court permit the development of long term care programs which would serve patients from the state hospitals at

---

16. R.A.J. v. Jones, "The Court Monitor's Second Report on the Board and Care Homes in Devine, Texas," June 1990.

17. R.A.J. v. Jones, "Defendant's Action Plan for Board and Care Homes in Devine, Texas," June 1990.

less expense than state hospital care. A task force was created to develop the concept of long term care and to address the question of whether the Court could support such a concept. The rationale for proposing the development of long term care programs was that approximately 45 percent of the patients in the state hospitals had resided there for over one year and one-half of that group resided there for over five years. As people were discharged from the hospitals over the years that rate has declined to approximately 35 percent who remain in the hospital beyond one year. In 1985, TXMHMR was proposing that 1,500 to 1,800 residents of the hospitals did not need the intensive programming of a psychiatric hospital and could be cared for in a different kind of residential facility. Staff suggested that these programs would need less rigorous standards than those set for psychiatric hospitals, thereby permitting the cost of the programs to be less. The value of this proposal was that the state might realize a savings of approximately $10 million per year by placing these patients in these facilities. During the task force process, the Review Panel asked questions about what kinds of staffing standards would be in place, what types of people would be served, what legal standards would be used to insure the protection of patients' rights, and what kind of treatment would be offered. The Panel also questioned whether patients would be committed to these facilities or would live there on a voluntary basis. After several meetings the Deputy Commissioner for Mental Health Services of TXMHMR decided that it would not be possible to come to agreement between the Defendants, the Review Panel, and the Plaintiffs about the program definitions and standards for such a program. He announced that the Defendants therefore would withdraw the proposal from the Court, stating that it would be possible for TXMHMR to accomplish its goals of placing people from inpatient long term care programs into community programs rather than by developing care programs under the jurisdiction of the R.A.J. Settlement Agreement.

TXMHMR's decision to withdraw the proposal was based largely upon its objection that the level of detail that the Review Panel was seeking inappropriately extended the authority of the Panel and Court into clinical decision making. The position of the Panel that clients had the protection of the Court and would remain under these protections when they went into other services was not specifically challenged by the state but it did cause the state to stop the pursuit of this idea.[18] The question about whether residents of extended care units could be served in less expensive programs did not go away and although it was debated periodically over the years it has not been adequately answered.

During 1986 there appeared to be several efforts to discharge sizeable numbers of clients from state hospitals. The most noticeable actions were the efforts to discharge geriatric clients from a facility with a predominantly geriatric population. These clients were discharged to local nursing homes. In addition, approximately 64 clients from an extended care unit at one hospital were placed in a long term care program in a nearby town and approximately 50 geriatric patients were moved from a state hospital to a program housed in a nursing home that proposed to specifically meet the special requirements of psychiatric patients by augmenting the services provided by the nursing home.

The placement of patients from the geriatric hospital were made over the objections of many of the hospital staff. The hospital staff believed that they were providing levels of care that the clients needed and that the care was superior to that provided by most nursing homes. Since many of these clients had resided in the hospital for 20 or more years they were concerned about the effects of the placement upon the coping capacities of the clients. During the winter of 1987, the Review Panel Coordinator traveled with TXMHMR staff from the Office of Clients' Rights and Protection to review nursing home placements which had taken place from the geriatric program. The reviewers observed a range of quality of care from high to mediocre to poor.

This was a striking finding since all nursing homes visited met the same Health Department standards and were funded by the same Medicaid reimbursement. It was apparent that nursing homes were not equipped to handle psychiatric clients. The attending physicians at the nursing homes were not psychiatrists and therefore were not specifically trained to deal with psychiatric symptoms and treatment. Many of the patients discharged from the hospitals to these homes did appear to fit into nursing homes because they had a level of physical and mental deterioration which was similar to that of other pa-

---

18. R.A.J. v. Miller, Joint Motion of Defendants, Plaintiffs, and the Review Panel to Withdraw Proposal to Establish Long Term Care Units, January 1986.

tients in the facilities. The fact that most of these clients were demented and that many other patients were also demented suggested that the settings were appropriate for most of the patients. However, these homes were not tolerant of disruptive behavior and patients were often overcontrolled by medications or restraints or were discharged back to the psychiatric hospital. Other patients gained or lost large amounts of weight in a short period of time. One did not receive needed medical care although the medical condition had been carefully documented in the hospital chart which had accompanied the client to the nursing home. The nursing home had chosen not to review the chart. Several clients did not seem to be involved in any kind of activities.

The level of psychiatric aftercare provided by the community mental health centers to these residents of nursing homes varied considerably. Several centers provided frequent reviews of clients, others did not provided any follow-up.

The Parties in the lawsuit resolved this issue in the same way they resolved the question of what constitutes adequate aftercare. They developed a set of procedures that mental health authorities should follow to provide follow-up to patients discharged from hospitals to nursing homes. Specifically, staff from the mental health authority should visit the nursing home to determine the appropriateness of the placement. The patient should visit the home prior to placement. Case workers must conduct two face-to-face contacts and two telephone contacts during the first two months after placement. Case workers must conduct at least one monthly contact thereafter. Monitoring of these procedures was conducted for several years until the Parties were convinced that the process was being adequately carries out.[19]

During 1986 Terrell State Hospital made a contract with a private nursing home provider and a community mental health center to provide services for all of the 64 residents of an extended care program at their state hospital. These patients were moved to a newly constructed facility in a rural community not far from the state hospital. The program represented an intensive, cooperative effort between the

---

19. R.A.J. v. Miller, Section 8: Stipulated Recommendations for Compliance, September 1987.

state hospital, a private nursing home provider, and the local community mental health center. The concept of the program was initially developed by the program director of the extended care unit at the state hospital. The state hospital funded the day-to-day placement of those patients who could not be funded by Medicare payments through their community services budget. The residential services and staffing were provided by the private provider and mental health aftercare services were provided by the local mental health center through a day program operated on the grounds of the facility. The facility was a modern nursing home building which was appropriately designed for the physical needs of this patient population.

The Review Panel Coordinator and two psychiatric consultants reviewed this program. They were impressed by the physical plant and by the enthusiasm and interest of the staff involved. The consultants however were concerned by the fact that the program was a locked facility and was in every way as restrictive as the state hospital extended care program. Although patients were not officially committed to this facility they were constrained to the facility. The rationale for locking was that the clients' functional capacities were such that they could not be trusted to leave the building on their own. The facility did face a busy highway and staff were concerned that if people left on their own that they could be injured on the highway. The Review Panel's consultants raised the question of whether the civil rights of the patients in this program were being violated and whether the program was actually operating as a hospital but not within the standards of a hospital.[20]

After discussing the consultants' concerns the state hospital and the program agreed that the door would be unlocked and that the program would operate as an open facility. The front door was unlocked though egress was monitored by a video camera and staff prohibited people from actually leaving the facility. The facility was obviously still concerned about security because of the functional capacity of their clients. There was the reality that many clients were so impaired that they would not be able to take care of themselves if they left the facility. The facility, therefore, was concerned about the program's relationship with the community if clients wondered

---

20. R.A.j. v. Miller, R.A.J. Review Panel Tenth Report to the Court, June 1987.

openly through the community. It was clear at this point that although doors were open that the facility intended to operate a closed, secure program.

A review in October 1990 revealed that the program had continued to keep its doors unlocked but that there was a high degree of staff supervision. The Monitor and his consultant were impressed that this program had matured over the years. There was greater comfort on the part of staff with the behaviors of the clients and there appeared to be less need to control clients than in the past. A psychiatric consultant had been hired by the facility and was providing weekly monitoring of medications. A program person was developing adequately individualized treatment plans and the program was providing appropriate psychosocial rehabilitation services.[21]

After the board and care homes in Medina County were scrutinized through the Monitor's reports and media coverage, one of the state hospitals invited the Monitor to look at board and care facilities that they were operating under their outreach department.

The Monitor and a psychiatric consultant went to Big Spring, Texas, in December 1990, to review board and care homes that receive clients referred by the outreach department of Big Spring State Hospital and to review the level of aftercare services that were provided to these clients by the outreach department of Big Spring State Hospital.

There were four board and care homes in Big Spring, Texas; two in Sweetwater, Texas; and one in Kermit, Texas. All of these homes are approved by the Big Spring State Hospital Outreach Department and meet their certification standards. These homes actively received referrals of clients by the hospital. The patients were all on the case load of the Big Spring State Hospital Outreach Department. The patients were supported by the clinics to participate in the day programs which were run by the outpatient department in the three different communities. Board and care providers were paid $22.00 a day per client for the board and care. This money was supplied through individual clients' SSI payments, personal funds, or if neither

---

21. R.A.J. v. Jones, The Court Monitor's Fourteenth Report to the Court, March 1991.

was sufficient, through financial support from the Big Spring State Hospital Outreach Department residential services budget.

The quality of the physical plants of the seven different board and care homes varied considerably. Several were considerably better than anything viewed in the Devine area. One facility included four homes. One was the provider's home with two clients, and the three other homes, all located next door to each other, had six clients each. All of these homes were well decorated and attractive, and clients had personal property in their rooms. This was something that was never seen in any of the Devine homes. Two homes were as physically barren as those seen in Devine. These buildings were at best marginally adequate.

An impressive part of the program for these clients was the coordinated care they received from Big Spring State Hospital Outreach Department. Each client was an active client with the Outreach Department Clinic, and each client was encouraged to participate in the psychosocial day program. The psychiatrist and the Monitor were both impressed by the fact that these clients were remarkably free of the symptoms of major mental illnesses. People were not hallucinating or preoccupied with their own delusions. They were well maintained on medications and appeared to be quite active.

A large number of clients were at the Corral, the psychosocial program operated in the town of Big Spring. This program ran a lawn maintenance service in the summer and an office janitorial service. It was therefore an active vocational program. Clients were at the day program cleaning it up after a Christmas party. The enthusiasm of both the clients and staff was noticeable. Day programs were also observed in the towns of Sweetwater and Kermit. The Monitor left these programs with the strong impression that this is what was meant by continuity of care and support by the mental health authority for people placed in the community. These programs were good examples of what the mental health system ought to be providing clients.

It was difficult to address questions of the adequacy of community aftercare through the requirements of the R.A.J. Settlement Agreement. This was largely because there was such conflict between the parties over the questions of the legitimacy of the Court's involvement in these issues. The State maintained that the Court had limited or no involvement in community aftercare issues although the initial jurisdiction was based upon the Settlement Agreement and subsequent actions of the Court. The State had originally agreed to the inclusion of adequate discharge plans. The State maintained however that there were no constitutional requirements to provide community services and the U.S. Justice Department supported this position. Defendants obviously did not welcome inquiry into community activities and were not able to view the Monitor as a consultant on these issues. Plaintiffs advocated for the broad provision of community services aimed at supporting clients from the hospitals in the community. The legal issues were never thoroughly explored through court hearings.

The broadest definitions of the adequacy of aftercare were provided through the negotiated criteria. Dr. Goldman's studies of these issues provided information about the provision of the five criteria.

Dr. Goldman found that the community mental health authorities were conducting assessments of clients referred from the hospitals, developing service plans and providing services at an acceptable level. Clients and advocates, however, did not accept these findings because they conflicted with their own experiences. So many people had experiences similar to those described by Genevieve Hearon, and they were aware of the lack of funding for community mental health services that they considered the Goldman Report findings as counterintuitive. The investigation of complaints led to some incremental examinations of community care issues. These examinations made the Defendants nervous because they were concerned that the Panel or Monitor was getting into new issues and might be broadening their roles. The examination of these issues did bring to light situations which had not been examined before. The incidents at Whisper Oaks brought up a question of whether this decision to discharge clients was done for clinical reasons or because of economic constraints. The exploration of the cottage industry of personal care homes in Devine brought to light the fact that there were many placements in fairly unregulated, stark settings and it was apparent that very few people in the field of mental health in the state knew anything about these programs. The examination of a secure nursing home program for the mentally ill also raised questions about how this type of program fit into a definition of community mental health services. All of these examples could be viewed as raising the question, Is this what we consider adequate care and want as community treatment?

If the criticism that the Review Panel or the Monitor created issues meant that at times situations people were previously unaware of were brought to light and questions were raised about the appropriateness of the situation, there was some validity to the criticism. Situations like the board and care homes had not been systematically examined and there was probably some value to a public examination of this situation.

Chapter 9

Evaluating Compliance with the Aftercare Standards

Howard H. Goldman and Anne Mathews Younes

Evaluation research played a key role in the R.A.J. case during the mid 1980's. Multiple case studies of institutions, based on personal inspections and interviews conducted in the early 1980's, gave way to empirical studies using standardized approaches to data collection. The empirical work focused on various remedies to the lawsuit, reflected in the Settlement, and the extent to which criteria for compliance with its standards had been met.

Just as the reach of the R.A.J. case and its Settlement Agreement extended beyond institutional walls to community services, so did the evaluations. Studies were conducted on the 35.50 incentive program for reducing the census of the state operated inpatient facilities and on the adequacy of the community-based system of mental health services. The most important studies, however, focused on compliance with the aftercare standards established to assure the quality of services for patients discharged from the state mental hospitals in the effort to achieve the staff-to-patient ratios required by the Settlement of the lawsuit.

This chapter provides some of the background, methods, and findings of the studies of compliance with the five supplemental aftercare criteria listed in Figure 1. The study reviewed the records of 700 patients discharged from Texas Department of Mental Health and Mental Retardation (TXMHMR) inpatient psychiatric facilities between January 1 and March 31, 1990. The supplemental criteria were established by the Court as part of the settlement of the R.A.J. v. Jones (previously R.A.J. v. Miller) class action suit. The material is taken from a series of reports to the R.A.J. Monitor and to the Court, based on research conducted between 1987 and 1990 by Howard Goldman and Anne Mathews Younes, assisted by several clinical raters and co-investigators, and by co-investigators, Catherine Jackson and Ann Skinner.

State Hospital Reform: Why Was It So Hard to Accomplish?

Figure 1
The Five Supplemental Criteria for
Community Based Aftercare Services

1. The MHA must make a good faith effort to make available and accessible those services specified in the community aftercare plans for patients discharged to their care for as long as the MHA determines that the client needs these services.

2. The LMHA will make a follow-up appointment for all persons referred for aftercare services and will document efforts made to assist the client in keeping the appointment.

3. The MHA will document outreach efforts made specifically in the effort to extend services specified in the community aftercare plan to hard to reach clients.

4. The MHA will make a good faith effort to make available case management services to those clients who qualify according to TXMHMR criteria.

5. The MHA will make a good faith effort to arrange for non-clinical support for patients in cases in which the Department's assessment indicates that long term hospitalization and chronicity of mental illness justify such action. This provision will apply only in those situations in which no other resources are available.

In 1987 the R.A.J. Monitoring Panel commissioned Drs. Goldman and Younes to conduct a study of compliance with the aftercare criteria in the cases of patients discharged from TXMHMR inpatient psychiatric facilities. In a report filed in February, 1988, they reviewed approximately 500 cases using a subjective scoring of each record on each of the five criteria (1=does *not* meet the standard, 2=minimally meets the standard, 3=meets the standard, 4=exceeds the standard). They found that 95% of the records were rated as 2–4 on criteria #1 and #2; 79% were rated 2–4 on criterion #3; 86% were 80 rated on criterion #4; and 72% were rated 2–4 on criterion #5.

Although the ratings were reliable, they were viewed as subjective. Overall, 22% of the ratings were scored as "2" or "minimally meets the standard." Defendants claimed that these cases met the standard; Plaintiffs felt that they did not. Evaluators felt that these ratings indicated that required services were not provided but that a good faith effort was made to provide them in the face of extenuating circumstances (e.g., "hard-to-reach" clients and severe resource limitations).

The evaluators, Monitor Panel, and Plaintiffs all concluded that the results of this investigation indicated that there was considerable room from improvement in the aftercare system in Texas. Defendants felt that the methodology was flawed and that the local mental health authorities (LMHAs) were held accountable to an unclear standard (operationalizing the aftercare criteria) without a clear explanation of expectations. In 1988 Judge Sanders ordered several changes in the criteria and asked for a new study. The Judge's Order suggested that the five aftercare criteria could serve as the basis for the evaluation, or the study could be done "...through the development of other criteria and methodology if the consultants so propose." The Monitor asked Dr. Goldman and Dr. Younes, again, to design and conduct the study.

The consultants decided to use the five criteria as the basis for the evaluation for conceptual, methodological, and practical reasons.

Conceptually, the criteria represent accepted measures of aftercare performance in Texas. They are face valid and touch upon important aspects of the aftercare of patients discharged from inpatient care. Although other areas of performance and other measures of adequacy of services might have been developed, the consultants felt unable to determine their specific relevance to the R.A.J. case.

Methodologically, prior experience indicated that the five criteria could be operationalized, especially following their clarification and revision, based on the prior evaluation. Using the five criteria also provided a benchmark of comparison and continuity with the prior study. Other criteria would have been more difficult to develop and operationalize, and there would be little assurance that the measures would be accepted as valid by the parties to the lawsuit. The consultants felt that involving the parties in the design of the evaluation was important to gain their support and understanding of the methodology. This was particularly true for the Defendants, as they had responsibility for explaining the study to the LMHAs and assisting in implementing the evaluation.

Practically, limitations in time and financial resources precluded developing and conducting a completely new methodology with new criteria. In particular, these limitations precluded the direct assessment of client needs and the outcomes of aftercare through in-person interviews or clinical evaluations. A direct assessment of the adequacy and quality of aftercare were also beyond the limitations of time and resources for this evaluation. Such investigations usually require an order of magnitude or greater resources than were available for the study.

A methodology based on a review of case records for performance on the five aftercare criteria was viewed as the best approach to the evaluation, given the advantages of this methodology under the constraints of limited time and resources. In the opinion of the consultants, a review of case records offered an acceptable method for assessing compliance with the five criteria of direct relevance to the R.A.J. v. Jones lawsuit, although it would not allow for a direct assessment of the quality of aftercare services, *per se*, and would not be a good method for determining if the needs of clients were being properly assessed. In spite of these limitations, the proposed methodology was considered to be an appropriate approach to the evaluation of aftercare in Texas.

During 1988 a preliminary methodology was developed in cooperation with the Defendants and the Plaintiffs, but there was difficulty operationalizing the concept of "good faith effort," which was central to the aftercare criteria. The Monitor asked for clarification from Judge Sanders, who stated that the Court would determine if there had been a "good faith effort," based on observations and opinions to be rendered by the evaluators. In 1989 the methodology was simplified and revised to create categories for clear compliance, clear non-compliance, and specific explanations for cases in which there were potentially extenuating circumstances. The basic methodology was finalized in August 1989 and was prepared for implementation.

Details of the basic methodology, agreed upon in August 1989, are beyond the scope of this chapter. However, it is important to explain how the issue of "good faith effort" and the documentation of compliance were handled. When evaluating a clinical record, there was a group of cases which obviously met the standard and another group that clearly did *not* meet the standard. There also was a group of cases where the standard was not completely met, but there was a documented explanation and evidence of attempts to overcome limitations. Cases in this group were considered to have been involved in a "good faith effort," as required by the standards. These cases partially met the standard and showed effort toward meeting the standard, even if performance was incomplete. Often resource limitations were noted as an explanation or barrier to implementation. The 1989 methodology differed from the original 1987 study in that explanations and efforts were documented for the judge to examine and upon which to base his final determination.

For example, with respect to criterion #2: The LMHA will make a follow-up appointment for all persons referred for aftercare services and will document efforts made to assist the client in keeping the appointment. The evaluators assessed the making of the appointment, the keeping of the appointment, efforts directed to assist clients, and explanations for failure to make or keep appointments or to provide assistance. Individuals who never kept an appointment were defined as "hard to reach" and were removed from further assessment. Individuals who were judged not to need aftercare services also were removed from the analysis.

A pilot test was conducted in the Fall of 1989 to assess the feasibility of implementing the methodology, to develop field procedures, and to design a form. A few categories were added to the basic methodology, based on this experience, and a form was developed to standardize the collection of data. In June 1989, Nancy Dittmar, Ph.D., of TXMHMR developed some data on discharges from the state hospitals during the first quarter of 1989 and suggested a sampling plan. For reasons of efficiency and cost-containment it was decided to sample 700 cases from three strata enabling the evaluation to find meaningful differences at the 95% confidence level.

It was decided to sample 250 records from the four large urban LMHAs (Austin, Dallas, Houston, and San Antonio) which accounted for 36% of the discharges in the first quarter of 1989. (Cases from Fort Worth were excluded from this stratum and included in another stratum because a large proportion of inpatients in the area are served at Fort Worth General Hospital and are not part of the R.A.J. class.) Two hundred records were to be sampled from the "outreach centers" operated by the state hospitals. These centers served small, typically rural, population centers, and were responsible for the aftercare of 21% of hospital discharges in early 1989. The remaining 250 discharges were to be sampled from those cases who were the responsibility of LMHAs with independent centers serving smaller cities and towns, suburban, and some rural areas. (Cases from Fort Worth were included in this stratum.) These LMHAs had contributed 43% of the total discharges in the 1989 survey.

Following the pilot test and agreement on the rating form in the Fall of 1989, TXMHMR conducted a training program for its LMHAs to explain the evaluation design, develop procedures, and prepare them for what would be expected in terms of performance and documentation. Special rating forms had been developed by TXMHMR for assessing the need for case management, non clinical support, and various other specified services.

The 700 records were sampled from discharges and furloughs from Texas state psychiatric hospitals during the first quarter of 1990 (January 1–March 31). Only clients who were reassigned to a LMHA were included in the sample. Each subject was identified to the LMHA ninety days after discharge or furlough. The relevant portions of the chart were then sent for rating with a cover sheet signed by the LMHA Chief Executive Officer (Superintendent, Director, or Executive Director) indicating that the records were complete and had not been altered. The ninety day period following discharge was the period of performance and rating, as specified in the evaluation methodology.

Charts were requested every two weeks beginning April 15 and ending on July 1, 1990 and were rated on an ongoing basis. All ratings were completed by the end of July 1990.

Rater training and reliability assessment began in April 1990. Two Masters-level psychiatric social workers had been previously hired to serve as raters of aftercare performance. They had been briefed on the R.A.J. case and the evaluation design. In April, two training sessions were held on the rating procedures and on the use of the scoring form. In May the first fifty records were available for rating. A consensus rating process was developed to achieve a high degree of inter-rater reliability from the outset of the study. The first ten records were read by the two social work raters, as well as by Dr. Goldman and Dr. Younes. Ratings on these records were done independently and then discussed until a consensus could be reached and standard rules for interpreting evidence could be developed. Twenty-five of the first fifty records were reviewed jointly and discussed by both social workers. Questions of interpretation and rating were also discussed with Dr. Younes, and any of the first fifty records which did not meet any one of the standards were sent to Dr. Goldman for additional review. The two social workers rated the remaining cases (c.650).

After the charts were received from the LMHA, they were randomly assigned to the social workers for review. When raters had questions, they often discussed their ratings with each other to achieve consensus. (The social workers eventually read 117 of each other's primary case assignments in an effort to improve reliability.) Furthermore, Dr. Younes reviewed every case in which there was a rating indicating possible non-compliance and a sample of the other records, checking for "false positive" ratings. She reviewed 293 records, including about eighty on which she was the sole reviewer.

The results of the chart reviews indicated the following: Nearly 80% of all of the 687 records reviewed had no deficiencies in any of the standards for aftercare set forth in this evaluation. Some of the 687 cases were removed from further analysis for a variety of reasons, e.g., patient died, moved from LMHA jurisdiction, or was otherwise hard to reach. With respect to the specific criteria:

Receipt of an appointment. Fewer than 3% (16/579) failed to meet the standard for criterion #2 (not receiving an appointment) and an equal number who received an appointment did not keep the appointment. Almost 95% (547/579) of cases met the standard for both aspects of criterion #2.

Development of a service plan and the attempt to provide the services. On criterion #1, 1.3% (6/481) of cases failed to meet the standard for developing an aftercare plan. A total of thirty-eight individuals (six cases evaluated on criterion #1 and thirty-two cases on criterion #2) either did not receive an appointment, did not keep an appointment and received no assistance to do so, or did not otherwise have an aftercare plan developed, and thus did not receive any aftercare services. Of those who had aftercare plans and were judged to need medication, 5.4% (17/316) did not meet the standard for medication management, 14.4% (31/215) of those recommended for the service did not meet the standard for psychosocial rehabilitation services, 22.7% (10/44) did not meet the standard for vocational rehabilitation, and 4.7% (4/86) did not meet the standard for residential services.

Case Management. On criterion #4, 15.6% (46/295) of cases did not receive case management services or did not receive appropriate evaluation. Resource limitation were cited in 21.7% (64/295) of cases, although substitute services were arranged for 14.5% (43/295) of all clients. Case management services posed a special problem for children and adolescents and for urban LMHA's.

Non-clinical Support Services. About 8.6% (44/512) of cases were not assessed for the need for non-clinical support on criterion #5, but once a need for housing, food, or clothing was identified, the LMHA virtually always made efforts to assist the client to meet those needs.

Outreach Efforts. Almost 14% (28/201) of the cases identified as needing outreach services did not receive them. Although all of the cases evaluated on criterion #3 were designated as "hard to reach", 85% (166/201) of them received outreach services, and resource limitations were identified in an additional 3% of cases.

Although LMHA's were offered the opportunity to identify resource limitations as a reason for failure to provide required services, this explanation was seldom offered unless accompanied by efforts to provide clients with substitute services.

The following conclusions were reported to the Monitor and the Court: This evaluation study indicates considerable compliance with the settlement of the R.A.J. case. In general, it was found that four out of five patients discharged or furloughed from the TXMHMR inpatient psychiatric facilities into the care of the LMHA's had no deficiencies detected on any of the five aftercare criteria. For the critically important criterion #2, compliance exceeded 95% for all but the "hard to reach" clients. For those clients referred into aftercare, almost 99% of them received an aftercare plan, as required in criterion #1. Overall, although there were thirty-eight cases in which the LMHA failed one of these five criteria, over 93% (n=541) of the 579 discharged patients considered on criterion #2 received aftercare appointments, kept those appointments, and had aftercare plans developed for them. For "hard to reach" clients, this study indicates that more than four out of five of them received outreach services (criterion #3).

With regard to actual receipt of services, the findings indicate that at least 85% of clients received identified services or substitutes for them. The data, however, also indicate that not many services were recommended in aftercare plans. Although 89% of 475 cases with aftercare plans were recommended for medication services, only 73% (349 cases) were recommended for outpatient services, and far fewer were recommended for psychosocial rehabilitation, 23% (109 cases), vocational rehabilitation, 20% (96 cases), and residential services, 24% (115 cases). Partial hospitalization services were specified so rarely that the data were not even analyzed. Overall performance on criterion #1 is enhanced because the aftercare service plans specify a need for few services, making it somewhat easier to deliver the specified services.

With regard to case management services assessed on criterion #4, 16% of clients failed to meet the standard. Case management services or substitutes were provided to 252 clients, less than 40% of the total sample. Although this may be all the case management that is required, it may also represent an under estimate of need. Such a determination is beyond the scope of the data reported in this study. A particular concern is the lack of case management services for children and adolescents and the problems urban areas have demonstrated in providing case management services to discharged patients. Case management services are the one area in which resource limitation were cited explicitly as a reason for failure to provide services.

The study found few problems with the provision of assistance in areas of non-clinical support. TXMHMR introduced a standard form for assessing the need for non-clinical support, which was used by the LMHA's 91% of the time. LMHA's provided assistance in almost every instance in which a need was identified.

Although the study found considerable compliance, it also found some room for improvement in almost all areas of performance, especially the provision of case management services and outreach to "hard to reach" clients. Furthermore, there is some concern that the aftercare plans recommend few services, although once identified, most needs are met with good faith effort, as defined in the study, between 85% and 95% of the time. Services for medication management are more likely to be delivered than outpatient, psychosocial, or vocational rehabilitation services. In particular, vocational rehabilitation services were delivered at the lowest rate of any service (77% of the time they were recommended).

There was considerable compliance with the aftercare criteria, especially the requirement to make appointments and conduct assessments for the development of aftercare plans, provision of case management services, and non-clinical support.

There were, however, a non-trivial number of clients (38) who did not receive appointments and aftercare plan. That is a serious deficiency, because failure to have an appointment upon discharge or an aftercare plan developed by a LMHA usually precludes the delivery of any aftercare services.

There continue to be deficiencies in the provision of case management services and outreach services could be improved, especially in the urban LMHA's. The need for case management services is recognized by the LMHA's, themselves, reflected in their explanations for the failure to provide services or for their need to provide substitute services.

Although the LMHA's deliver services to between 85%-95% of clients in every category of clinical need and almost all clients in the categories of non-clinical need, the LMHA's tend to recommend fewer services than expected. In our judgment, this reflects a limited array of aftercare services available in most areas in Texas, which leads to lowered expectations and limited aftercare plans. This judgment is based upon the comparison of the Texas data with related data from the Robert Wood Johnson Foundation Program on Chronic Mental Illness evaluation, on the prior study of aftercare services in Texas, and on professional judgments formed during the review of the case records. Only a more detailed study of client needs, derived from a more detailed data base and probably including clinical interviews, would answer the questions that remain about the adequacy of the assessment of client needs in Texas.

The findings of a decline in performance over the ninety day period of the study indicates that repeated evaluations and monitoring of the aftercare services would likely improve record keeping and the adequacy of the aftercare services in Texas.

Having demonstrated the ability to achieve considerable compliance with the five supplemental aftercare criteria, in spite of limited resources, TXMHMR should continue to improve the availability of services in its aftercare system. The serious deficiencies noted in the area of case management services and the continued need to improve outreach services should be corrected. The general level of aftercare services appears to be minimally adequate, at best, and needs improvement in the availability of specialized services such as psychosocial and vocational rehabilitation, as well as residential services.

The Monitor should continue to oversee an ongoing process of evaluation and monitoring of aftercare services in Texas. This study methodology, or a similar study method, should be conducted on a recurrent basis, without specific warning or special preparation by the LMHA's. Repeated evaluation is needed to assure continued compliance with aftercare criteria and other standards and to monitor for any improvements that signaled that ongoing monitoring would be required.

The Texas Department leadership understood the need to internalize this evaluation. Their commitment to maintaining the standards and evaluating their efforts were promising and exemplary. This commitment might not have been achieved without the close collaboration between the Monitor, his evaluators, and the defendants' own evaluation and quality assurance group, during the design phase of the evaluation. The independence of the clinical assessments of compliance was required to assure the validity of the findings, but the collaboration was essential to the ongoing success of the enterprise of improving care for the plaintiff's class and for all individuals with severe mental illness in Texas.

Chapter 10

Politics and Costs

David Pharis

Although the R.A.J. lawsuit primarily involved the attorneys for the Parties—the staff of the Texas Department of Mental Health and Mental Retardation (TXMHMR) and the Review Panel or Monitor representing the federal court—in a broader sense the lawsuit was the concern of the governor, state legislators, mental health advocates, and a variety of people who were interested and concerned about public policy. The lawsuit created public policy which in turn generated political reactions. Governmental leaders were acutely concerned about the interventions of a federal judge. They were concerned that such interventions would interfere with their responsibilities and capacity to perform their functions as legislators. The state agency was obviously concerned about its autonomy in performing its duties. All of these actors were concerned about the cost of the lawsuit in terms of both the administrative costs of the monitoring mechanism and the cost that requirements of the lawsuit could place upon the TXMHMR's budget.

The Review Panel and later the Court Monitor became convinced that TXMHMR's operating budget was inadequate to support the requirements of the lawsuit. TXMHMR was very reluctant to have the Review Panel advocate for increased operating budgets. The agency correctly interpreted that their role was to seek funding but they were concerned that drawing attention to the needs of the lawsuit could cause negative reactions on the part of the legislature. The Review Panel and then the Monitor, however, felt that they had an ongoing responsibility to advocate for adequate funding.

Conflicts around perceived interference on the part of the Court and its monitoring mechanism in the life of both the legislature and the state agency and concerns about administrative costs of the lawsuit and the adequacy of the TXMHMR operating budget persisted throughout the life of this lawsuit. This chapter will discuss the interplay of these concerns upon the activities of the actors in this situation.

Adequate funds for the requirements of the lawsuit and the administrative costs of the lawsuit were always important issues in this case. The fact that the state was required to pay for administrative costs of the suit and was expected to adequately fund requirements of the lawsuit was an ongoing irritant to the state legislature and the source of conflict between the parties in the suit. The 1981 Settlement Agreement ended with the statement:

> The Commissioner and other Defendants as appropriate, including the Texas Board of Mental Health and Mental Retardation, shall make every effort within the law of Texas to obtain appropriate budgetary authorization from the Texas legislature in an amount sufficient to insure the fulfillment of the requirements of this Settlement Agreement.
>
> Defendants shall make proper and timely application for any and all funding sources available from state, local, or federal governments for programs affected by this settlement.[1]

In addition, the State of Texas was expected to pay the Plaintiffs' attorneys fees and fund an annual operating budget for the Review Panel and the subsequent Court Monitor's compliance monitoring activities. Plaintiffs' attorneys submitted retroactive billing on a quarterly basis. The Court Monitor submitted six-month projected budget requests at the beginning of each fiscal year and once the budget was approved by the Parties and the Court, received monies for two six-month operating budgets. Both the Plaintiffs' attorneys fees and the Monitor's operating budget were funded through a General Revenue Fund. This mechanism was revised during the 1995 legislative session and the attorneys fees and the Monitor's budget have been charged to TXMHMR's operating budget since that time.[2]

The cost of funding lawsuit requirements as well as the costs of funding the administrative mechanisms of this suit were also a source

---

1. R.A.J. v. Kavanagh, Settlement Agreement, April 1981, p. 28.

2. State of Texas Appropriations Bill, 74th Legislative Session, Austin, Texas, September 1995.

Politics and Costs 195

of conflict between the Parties and the Legislature. The Legislature disliked federal interventions because it interpreted such interventions as interference in the legislature's powers of policy and fiscal decision making.[3] John Sharp, the Texas Comptroller of Public Accounts, raised the question of who is running state government—the Legislature or the courts—in an article entitled "Calling the Shots: Lawsuits Help Define State Spending,"[4] Sharp states:

> None of the Court orders has dictated how much money the state should spend to upgrade services, but the far-ranging decrees certainly have complicated the budget writing process. Of the typical biennial appropriations bill, budget analysts estimate about 9 percent is devoted to responding to Court orders. Another 17 percent is tied to formula-driven spending; 58 percent is earmarked for expenditures required by the constitution or state statutes. That leaves only 16 percent of spending that is discretionary, allowing lawmakers to exercise flexibility in making budgetary cuts or expansions.[5]

The philosophical question about activist courts intervening in the legislative business was intensified in Texas due to the fact that during the 1970's there were federal cases filed against the Texas Department of Criminal Justice,[6] the Texas Youth Commission,[7] and TXMHMR for both its state hospitals and state schools.[8] [9] In addition, there was a federal case involving the adequacy of school financing.[10] Each of these cases involved years of litigation and the implementation of a settlement phase which required extensive funding by the Legislature. Each case should be judged on its own merits but the fact that there have been so many cases in this state may suggest

---

3. Perez, A., *Major Litigation against the States: Policy Recommendations on Dealing with the Issues*. Master's Degree Professional Report, The L.B.J. School of Public Affairs, Austin, Texas, 1994.

4. Sharp, J., *Calling the Shots: Lawsuits Help Define State Spending*, Texas Comptroller of Public Accounts, Austin, Texas, 1992.

5. Ibid.

6. Ruiz v. Estelle, 1980.

7. Morales v. Turman.

8. R.A.J. v. Gilbert, 1974.

9. Lelsz v. Kavanagh, 1974.

10. Edgewood v. Kirby, 1989.

something about the state's attention to the vulnerable issues of human services.

During the period from 1982 through 1995, Texas ranked from 49th through 42nd in the nation in terms of per capita expenditures for mental health services. E. F. Torrey in his three reports titled *Care of the Seriously Mentally Ill—A Rating of State Programs* not only ranked the merit of state programs programmatically based on his own subjective judgments, but also presented public mental health expenditure data from which he drew conclusions about the adequacy of funding.[11] In the Second Edition, based on 1985 expenditure data, Texas was ranked 49th in the nation in terms of per capita expenditures for mental health services. At the same time, however, the state ranked 22nd in terms of per capita income. Torrey suggested from this that the state could clearly choose to fund mental health services more adequately.[12] The 1990 report, based upon 1987 expenditure data, again ranked Texas as 49th in the nation in per capita spending for mental health services. Torrey constructed a generosity index representing the number of cents each state spends on mental health per $100 of per capita income. The higher the index, the more generous the state. The highest rank on this index was 78 with several states ranking in the 40's and 30's. Texas was ranked as 15 on this generosity index.[13] Torrey editorialized that the appropriations certainly reflected the will of the legislature and a lack of interest in the mentally ill. The National Association of State Mental Health Program Directors, in a publication presenting 1993 expenditure data, ranks Texas as 42nd in per capita mental health expenditures with a rate of $31.48. New York is ranked second with a rate of $130.94 per capita expenditure and the United States average is $54.21. It is interesting that Texas ranks fifth among the states in terms of total mental health expenditures whereas New York ranks first. For per capita mental health state hospital expenditures, Texas ranked 36th with a per capita rate of $18.69 with a national average of $28.57. For per capita expenditures in community mental health

---

11. Torrey, E.F., Wolfe, S.M., Flynn, L.M., *Care of the Serious Mentally Ill: A Rating of State Programs*. A Joint Publication of Public Citizen Health Research Group and the National Alliance for the Mentally Ill. Washington, DC, First Edition 1986, Second Edition 1988, Third Edition 1990.

12. Ibid., Second Edition 1988.

13. Ibid., Third Edition 1990.

programs, Texas ranked 39th with a per capita expenditure of $11.48 and a national average of $24.24.[14]

In 1981, the state hospital budgets totaled $128.3 million and contracted community services $48.5 million. The total mental health budget for that year was $177.2 million. In 1995, the state hospital budgets had grown to $230.4 million, an 85 percent increase, while the contracted community services was $252.5 million for a 439 percent increase over the 1981 budget. The total mental health budget for 1995 was $519.3 million for a 196 percent increase over the 1981 mental health budget. These figures are not adjusted for inflation (see Appendix I).

The Court never issued any specific orders with a fiscal note attached; however, many Court orders did require specific funding. The fire safety renovations and the staff ratio line items are examples of major expenditures based on lawsuit requirements. From 1981 through 1990, when most of the fire safety code issues had been brought into compliance with the requirements of the lawsuit, $137.4 million had been appropriated by the Legislature to meet the life safety code requirements. In 1986 through 1989, $73.2 million were appropriated by the Legislature to meet the staff ratio requirements of the lawsuit. Much of this money was placed in community services through the $35.50 Program. All this money was specifically generated by requirements of the lawsuit. Other budgetary growth is less easy to track because it was put in the budget under the general auspices of R.A.J. funding. The growth of community services, outside of the framework of the $35.50 Program is an example of this. Other than the money transferred to community centers through the $35.50 Program, growth could not be specifically identified as connected to R.A.J. requirements. However, there probably was an increase of appropriations due to the focus that the lawsuit was placing upon community services.

TXMHMR did develop a funding formula for its state hospitals that purported to adequately fund JCAHO and R.A.J. requirements. The funding formula allocated for professional and attendant staff based upon the acuity levels of a group of 30 clients. Acute services, children's units, and other intensive psychiatric services required

---

14. Lutterman, T., Funding Sources and Expenditures of State Mental Health Agencies. National Association of State Mental Health Program Directors, Washington, DC, 1995.

richer staffing than some other programs. The Monitor trusted this funding formula and during the legislative sessions in 1988–1995 maintained that funding according to this formula should produce adequate staffing to meet the Court's requirements. He believed that funding through this formula would bring adequate resources to the hospital system so that questions of compliance could become questions of management and performance rather than resource adequacy.

Although the Court never issued specific orders with a fiscal note attached, Judge Barefoot Sanders did examine the powers of the Court to enforce its orders:

> Having found that Defendants are not complying with several portions of the Agreement, the Court must determine an appropriate remedy. The Court reserves this determination pending the receipt of recommendations from the Plaintiffs, Defendant TXMHMR, the United States, and the Panel.

> Without limiting or foreclosing any appropriate suggestions which the parties may advance, the Court notes the following options available to it:

> 1. Appointment of a Special Master to oversee and direct Defendants' efforts to achieve compliance with the Court's decree;

> 2. Discharging some patients from the hospitals to resolve the inadequacies in patient-staff ratios;

> 3. Requiring compliance by a date certain, with express penalties for failure to comply.

> The Court is aware of the serious implications posed by some of the foregoing. Nevertheless, the Court is obligated to enforce its judgment. That is especially true in this case where commitments, voluntarily made by Defendants in the Settlement Agreement, are not being honored.

> A federal court possesses a broad range of equitable powers available to enforce and effectuate its orders and judgments. *See, e.g., Gates v. Collier*, 616 F.2d 1268 (5th Cir. 1980), *reh'g denied en banc*, 641 F.2d 403 (5th Cir. 1981); *New York State Association for Retarded Children*

v. Carey, 596 F.2d 27 (2d Cir. 1979), *cert. denied*, 444 U.S. 836 (1979); *United States v. City of Detroit*, 476 F. Supp. 512 (E.D.Mich. 1979). *See also, Wyatt v. Stickney*, 325 F. Supp. 781 (M.D.Ala. 1971), *supplemented at* 344 F. Supp. 387 (M.D.Ala. 1972).[15]

The Judge also occasionally focused attention on the adequacy of funding:

> Compliance by Defendants with the requirements of the Settlement Agreement, and court orders (including Recommendations) related thereto, will end this litigation. Defendants have substantially complied in some areas, and the Court has ordered reduced monitoring, with the goal of dismissal. However, it appears from the history of this case that Defendants have never been provided sufficient funds for complete compliance. Unless provided adequate funds by the Legislature, Defendants will never achieve compliance, and this lawsuit will never end.[16]

The Texas Legislature meets every other year during the odd numbered years from January through May. During this time it develops a two-year budget for the years beginning the following September 1. During the progress of the R.A.J. lawsuit, legislators claimed that court involvement in a state agency's activities interfered with their legislative-policy and fiscal-priority decision making. The Court Monitor never sensed a lack of legislative power since he experienced each legislative session as a struggle over whether there would be adequate funds to meet the requirements of the lawsuit. The legislative decision making process followed a routine process of submission of an agency budget request based upon directions of the legislature. These directions usually included three levels of funding—the current funding level, a percentage increase over that, and a "wish list" request. The budget request was reviewed by the Legislative Budget Board which made a formal recommendation. This recommendation was then reviewed by both the State House of Representatives and the Senate. Separate recommendations from the House and Senate could then be reconciled through a joint reconciliation committee with final recommendations to both bodies. The Governor's Office

---

15. R.A.J. v. Miller, Memorandum Opinion and Order, April 1984, pp. 19–20.

16. R.A.J. v. Jones, Memorandum Opinion and Order, September 1989, p. 20

could submit a budget which would play an advisory role in the legislative negotiation process.

The following excerpt from the R.A.J. Review Panel's Tenth Report to the Court illustrates the nature of the struggle for adequate funding.

> The 1988–89 legislative budget request represented approximately a 15% increase above the 1987 level of funding. In terms of the mental health portion of the budget this request was aimed primarily at meeting requirements of the R.A.J. Settlement Agreement and at further developing community services. The Review Panel considered this budget request to be minimally adequate for compliance with the Settlement Agreement. The overall request was as follows:
>
> The 1987 budget total for TXMHMR had been $635.8 million.
>
> - The 1988 request from TXMHMR was $782.2 million.
>
> - The 1989 request was $756.8 million.
>
> - The Legislative Budget Board recommended $650 million for 1988 and $637.7 million for 1989.
>
> - The House Appropriations Bill recommended $677.6 million for 1988, which was $104.6 million less than the 1988 request. They recommended $674.3 million for 1989 which was $82.5 million less than the request.
>
> - The Senate Appropriations Bill recommended $724.9 million for 1988 which was $57.2 million less than the request and $693.5 million for 1989 which was $63.3 million less than the budget request.

From 1981 through 1990, when most of the fire safety code issues had been brought into compliance with the requirements of the lawsuit, $137.4 million had been appropriated by the legislature to meet the life safety code requirements. In 1986 through 1989, $73.2 million were appropriated by the legislature to meet the staff ratio requirements of the lawsuit. Much of this money was placed in community services through the $35.50 Program. All this money was specifically generated by requirements of the lawsuit.

The TXMHMR budget request was not based upon an expansive request to fully develop the six year plan but rather was a narrow, focused attempt to increase community services and bring the hospitals into compliance with the requirements of the lawsuit. The budget request was based upon assumptions that the censuses in the hospitals would continue to decrease over the biennium and the adequacy of the request was highly dependent upon the correctness of this assumption and upon good management and leadership in the facilities.

The primary compliance issues which need to be addressed through the budget request are the staffing requirements in the facilities, new JCAHO requirements for increased doctor and nursing coverage, monitoring from Central Office of placements in the communities, and the development of community based mental health services. The majority of the new money in Defendants' request goes for the development of community services.

TXMHMR requested $73.6 million for capital improvements and life safety code renovations in the institutions. $15.6 million of this was specified for life safety code renovations in the state hospitals and the state schools. The additional requests were aimed at addressing maintenance and upkeep the physical plants of the institutions, roadways, and in other major maintenance items.

In 1987 the operating costs of the state hospitals was $180.8 million. For 1988 TXMHMR requested $193.0 million or $12.2 million over the 1987 level and in 1989 TXMHMR requested $196.9 or $16.1 million over 1987. Neither the House nor the Senate came close to the budget request for the state hospitals and recommended levels which were lower than the 1987 budget level. The House recommended a budget of $171.8 million or $9 million lower for 1988 and $166.7 million or $13.1 million lower for 1989. The Senate recommended $175.3 million for 1988, which is $5.5 million lower than the current operating budget and for 1989 the Senate recommended $172.2 million or $10.6 million lower than the current operating budget. The Senate did recommend $3.5 million more for this line item than the house. It is the Panel's understanding that the TXMHMR budget increases for the hospitals were intended to accomplish two things: (1) to fund the increased demands for staffing of psychiatrists and nurses in the hospitals placed by revised JCAHO accreditation standards and (2) to provide additional monies to develop community based services which are funded by the outreach departments of the eight state hospitals. These services have been historically underfunded. In the Review Panel's opinion neither the House or Senate recommendations adequately fund these two items. The assumption that the censuses of the state hospitals will continue to decline and therefore permit an increased level of services for those remaining in the hospitals is an unproven assumption. If this assumption proves to be false, the funding would be grossly inadequate.

The 1987 funding for contracted community services was $72.3 million. The TXMHMR budget request for 1988 was $83.1 million and in 1989 was $94.0 million. The House and Senate actually both agreed on increasing the funding of this line item and both are recommending $87.0 million for 1988 which is a $14.7 million increase over the 1987 level and $96.6 million for 1989 which is a $24.3 million increase over the 1987 level. These monies can certainly be anticipated to increase the number of services in the community mental health system.

A March version of the Governor's budget for 1988–89 depicted a $67.4 million decrease from the 1987 operating budget for TXMHMR. This included $26 million from the mental health budget. The Panel considered that this budget would make it impossible to comply with the requirements of the lawsuit.

A meeting was arranged between the Governor, the Coordinator of the Review Panel, and the Expert Consultant in the Lelsz case to discuss compliance issues of the two court cases and the need for adequate funding for compliance.

This meeting took place early in April 1987. The participants of the meeting were the Governor, two Court Monitors, the chairman of the TXMHMR board, and attorneys for the Governor. There was a frank discussion of the compliance issues of the two cases. The two monitors presented their position that the 1988–89 TXMHMR budget request was only minimally adequate for compliance with the two cases. Beyond that statement there was no actual discussion about budget figures in the meeting. The Governor stated, however, that there would not be funding below the 1987 current budget and that the only question would be whether there could be additional funding. Since that time the Review Panel has become aware that the Governor has mentioned in news conferences that this meeting took place and has said that he considers his budget adequate for compliance with the lawsuits. At this point the Panel is unclear as to what the Governor's budget proposal for TXMHMR is. The importance of a Governor's budget is primarily the influence it can have upon the negotiations between the House and Senate Committees and the Conference Committee. A Governor's budget would also be very relevant if a governor were to ever veto line items in an agency's budget.

At this point, however, the conference committee between the House and the Senate is still working on a resolution between the House and Senate proposals. The Review Panel maintains its analysis that the budget request from TXMHMR was minimally adequate to fund compliance with this court case. Neither the House nor the Senate recommendations fully meet this budget request. The Senate Appropriations Bill comes closest to funding the full request but there are serious gaps in funding which may make compliance impossible. These are in the areas of program administration where approximately $700,000 underfunding may make it difficult to conduct needed compliance monitoring. A $17.6 million cut for 1988 and a $26 million cut for 1989 from the proposed hospital budgets will impair meeting the JCAHO accreditation standards and will seriously impair the hospital outreach departments developing needed community based aftercare services. A $3.7 million reduction in the operating cost of Harris County Psychiatric Hospital from the budget request may slow down the operation of that facility and decrease the impact of that community, hospitals upon the delivery system in the Houston area. Cuts in the budgets for both Tarrant County Psychiatric Hospital and the Human Development Centers may have the same effect upon the service delivery in their own areas. The most positive result of the appropriation process has been the $39 million which has been placed into contracted community services. This will definitely have great impact upon the mental health centers' capacity to serve patients in the community.

At this point (May 1987) it seems very probable that there will not be an appropriations bill from the regular session of the 70th Legislature and that in fact it will be necessary to have a special session of the legislature in the summer of 1987. The appropriation levels of the House and Senate will remain to be decided during that session and the actions of the Governor will also remain to be decided. The needs of Texans for adequately funded mental health services will not go away and the needs for adequate funding for compliance with the court cases will not diminish. The fact is that in order to meet the requirements of the suit there must be an adequate appropriation from the legislature. At this point the problems have not been resolved and the Review Panel will continue to monitor the legislative process and will report to the Court upon the adequacy of the appropriations.[17]

In his professional report, *Major Litigation against the States: Policy Recommendations on Dealing with the Issues*, Arturo Perez identified that at the time of his research in 1994 forty states were involved in federal law suits concerning the adequacy of school funding, all but four states had federal and state law suits in their adult and juvenile criminal justice systems, and at least 27 states were involved with law suits in their state school and state hospital programs. All federal cases involved the question of a violation of consti-

---

17. R.A.J. v. Miller, Tenth Report to the Court, May 1987, pp. 61–66.

tutional rights. Perez examined the question of whether federal court intervention interfered with the legislature's policy and financial decision-making responsibilities. Most legislators maintained that court involvement certainly interrupted the legislative process. Advocates for plaintiffs maintained that court involvement was only necessary when legislative actions had created situations which violated constitutional rights. Action or inaction in such instances had created a situation which was a violation of constitutional protections requiring court remedies.

Perez reviewed the literature on federal court intervention and studied several cases in depth during which he interviewed judges, court monitors, attorneys, and state legislators for several selected cases. The R.A.J. case was one of his study cases and he therefore interviewed many of the actors in this case. Perez illustrated through his description of interviews that most legislators resented federal intervention and saw it as strongly interfering with their responsibility for policy and priority setting. Advocates on the other hand saw federal interventions as a last-ditch effort to provide remedies for classes of disenfranchised people who were not adequately attended to by representation.[18]

There is no question that litigation takes an issue out of the usual legislative process which is run through voting, lobbying, and advocacy from constituents. Legislators maintain that they represent the will of their constituents and they can justify funding decisions and other priority policy decisions as representing the will of these constituents. A lack of focus on a particular group therefore can be interpreted as a representation of the priority placed on that issue or group by the general population. The introduction of issues through litigation certainly alters this process. If there are determinations of violations of state or federal policy, the Court can intervene, order remedies, and issue sanctions, placing a whole new infrastructure upon the state legislative process. Legislators would argue that advocates learn to manipulate the legislative process. On the other hand, advocates would probably maintain that their clients (the mentally ill, mentally retarded, inmates of the criminal justice system) are disenfranchised classes of people who have little or no influence upon

---

18. Perez, *Major Litigation against the States*, pp. 20–25.

the legislative process. Therefore, their only recourse is litigation (see Appendices II and III).

A case like R.A.J. v. Gilbert is complicated when there is no initial finding of fact. The case was settled out of court with the state not admitting to violations of constitutional rights. This can create a situation where Defendants say that they will make changes but at the same time can maintain that problems were not so great in the first place. This situation makes it difficult to objectify questions of fact.

The positions of the actors in class action litigation often become polarized. Advocates for their plaintiffs may maintain that there group is powerless or placed in a situation where their needs are not met. Legislators can maintain that the use of litigation is a means of circumnavigating the usual legislative process and undermines this process. The legislators perceive that advocates try to accomplish agendas through the court process which they have not been able to sell through the legislative process. Litigation therefore takes the place of lobbying. The administrators of a state agency may maintain the adequacy of their programs and therefore the incorrectness or the lack of validity of the litigation. They may therefore fight implementation of the suit or they may recognize validity of the issues of the suit and work toward correcting inadequacies. If they do validate the issues they may run the risk of being seen by the legislature as using the courts to put pressure upon the legislature for funding. The court monitors or the courts themselves, if they believe that there is validity to reported violations and subsequent remedies, can be expected to advocate for compliance with the court ordered remedies.

Perez interviewed Judge Sanders about his thoughts about the R.A.J. and Lelsz litigation. The following is Perez's summary of this interview:

> Sanders stated that the state could have avoided many years of litigation over its programs for the mentally ill and mentally retarded had it simply provided sufficient monies for operating the programs of the Texas Department of Mental Health and Mental Retardation. By choosing not to provide adequate levels of funding for these programs, Sanders said he had no other option but to rule that the state had failed to meet its own constitutional requirements. He also added that any state legislature seeking to avoid the pitfalls of litigation could carry out the obliga-

tions that the state had agreed to, whether in corrections, education, or other programs.

Sanders adds that money will not solve everything but that it can go a long way towards solving the problems that are found in state programs. He believes that states can avoid litigation if they are willing to look forward and avoid violations of the constitution, anticipating that money will be needed, and providing adequate level funding. He says this is a key to avoiding a situation where litigation is the only option left open for advocates. His review of the relationships between the legislature and the judiciary is that the remedies that the courts prescribe may require additional allocation of funds but that the courts are not taking away any powers from the legislators. He contends that the settlements that are reached in many of the major cases against the state are reminders of the ways in which state institutions or programs should properly operate. As an impartial player in the process he does not believe that he should give any consideration to the amount of money that will be required by the state to correct the problems in its programs.

Judge Sanders believes that if legislators have a problem with the judiciary because of the process of litigation is outside of the normal process of lobbying the legislators have learned to work with regarding special interest. Sanders views those who have no political power as being only able to assert themselves through the courts and this conflicts with the way the system of lobbying operates. He observes that legislators will understandably have a problem when advocates circumvent the legislative process and seek a solution by going to the courts or using the threat of going to the courts. But, he also assumes that legislatures must face the realities of state commitments to the mentally ill and mentally retarded as well as others that are reliant on state services, care, or protection.[19]

---

19. Perez, *Major Litigation against the States*, p. 12. From telephone interview between Arturo Perez and Judge Barefoot Sanders, Chief United States District Judge, Northern District of Texas, July 22, 1993.

Administrators of the Texas Department of Mental Health and Mental Retardation often felt caught between the pressures of the Court and the reactions of the Texas legislature. During the early years of implementation of the lawsuit it was clear that the Commissioner and other chief policy makers did not want to imply in any way that funding was inadequate to meet the requirements of the suit. Messages from the TXMHMR administration were always that they would do the best they could with what they had and that that should be acceptable to meet Court requirements. Administrators appeared very reluctant to identify the need for funding from the legislature for requirements of the lawsuit because they were concerned that the legislature would react negatively to any mention of federal intervention. Dr. Gary Miller, the TXMHMR Commissioner from 1982–1988, persistently maintained that TXMHMR was doing everything they could to comply with the requirements of the case, were in fact complying with Court requirements, and were within the top ten mental health departments in the nation in terms of quality of care. He recognized Texas' national funding rank and took credit for excellent management within tight budgetary constraints. Dr. Miller publicly stated that the agency was doing everything it could to achieve appropriate financing and then publicly stated that the agency would perform adequately within the constraints of the legislative appropriations.

Dr. Miller clearly disagreed with the findings of the Review Panel. He eloquently expresses his antipathy with the Court's involvement in his chapter titled "Reform Through Litigation: A Commissioner's Perspective." Dr. Miller's beliefs about the lawsuit publicly expressed in the document "Living Under Lawsuits," was clearly more antagonistic and adversarial than the attitude expressed by his successor Dennis Jones.[20] Mr. Jones maintained that he agreed with the objectives of the lawsuit and wanted to work cooperatively with the plaintiffs and the Court Monitor to achieve those objectives. He also began to make clear statements in his budget requests about the need for increased levels of services and would make diplomatically stated assessments of the negative effects of budget cuts and restrictions.

During each legislative session the Court asked that the Court Monitor present an analysis of the adequacy of TXMHMR's budget request

---

20. Miller, G. E.; "Living Under Lawsuits", Memorandum to all employees of the Texas Department of Mental Health and Mental Retardation, Austin, Texas, July, 1987

and the subsequent legislative responses to this request and make recommendations about the adequacy of these actions to meet the requirements from the lawsuit. During several legislative sessions, the Court conducted a conference during the latter part of the legislative session to discuss the possible implications of proposed funding actions. These conferences were public and were reported upon by the media. The Court never issued court orders about the adequacy of legislative actions. The Monitor did consider it his responsibility to meet with the legislative leaders and testify to the legislative committees in order to advocate for adequate funding of lawsuit requirements.

As the lawsuit continued year after year, legislators became increasingly negative to the suit. They became convinced by 1992 that the court case was a black hole in which they could deposit funds and from which there would be no positive conclusion. This idea was actively circulated by TXMHMR administrators. During the 1993 legislative session Commissioner Dennis Jones was criticized by members of the legislature for having participated in a court conference on the adequacy of legislative actions during the present session where he discussed implications of possible funding actions. Legislators reportedly accused him of participating in the Court's pressure for the legislature to fund according to the Court's wishes.

During the 1991 and 1993 legislative sessions the legislature did fund the hospitals at the funding formula level that both TXMHMR and the Court Monitor considered adequate to meet JCAHO and R.A.J. requirements. The funding at this level and the implementation of the 1992 Settlement Agreement, which focused upon measuring compliance through an agreed upon measurement system, led the hospitals to ultimately comply with the lawsuit's standards.

It is somewhat difficult to calculate accurate costs of the administrative portion of the lawsuit because calculations for the attorneys' fees and the Monitor's Office come from different sources. The Comptroller's Office kept track of appropriations to both the Monitor's Office and the Plaintiffs' attorneys but did not separate the expenditures. The Monitor's Office kept accounts of costs during the history of the operation of the office. Its accounting, however, reflects actual expenditures.

Sharp reports that the combined costs of Plaintiffs attorneys and the Court Monitor in the R.A.J. case from its inception until April

1992 was $3.1 million.[21] Application for attorneys fees since April 1992 to September 1996 was an additional $240,355. The Court Monitor's Office records indicate that from January 1982 through February 1992 the office spent $2.1 million. From February 1992 through September 1996, the office spent an additional $1.5 million. An attempt at reconciling the Comptroller's figures with office accounts of the Court Monitor would suggest that the Court Monitor's Office from 1982 through September 1996 has expended $3.6 million. There was an additional amount of $3.3 million in Plaintiff's attorneys fees. This would suggest that the administrative costs of this lawsuit from its inception in 1974 through September 1996 has been approximately $7 million.

This lawsuit remained political in most senses of the word. Realities, as demonstrated by the different opinions expressed by the Commissioners and myself, in this case often remained subjective realities of the beholder. Dr. Mechanic, in his Forward and Afterward, recognizes the conflict between the actors in this case and acknowledges the turmoil that staff suffered while the parties struggled with each other. He also points out correctly that the administrative costs, $7 million, does not take into account any of the social costs of this case. In his Memorandum Opinion and Order dated October 14, 1997, Judge Sanders dismissed the R.A.J. v. Gilbert litigation from the jurisdiction of the Court. He stated in part:

> The controversies which constantly erupted between 1981 and 1990 resulted, in general, from sharply differing interpretations of the 1982 Agreement and allegations of Defendants' lack of compliance. The Court held a number of evidentiary hearings on these disputes and issued several rulings. However, by 1991, it was clear that the litigation was becoming increasingly contentious and likely to become more so. No end was in sight. At the Court's direction the Monitor, Plaintiffs, and Defendants entered into extensive discussions which resulted in a new agreement—the 1992 Settlement Agreement, approved by the Court March 24, 1992. That Agreement sets forth the method and conditions for dismissal of this case. *See* Agreement at 26.

---

21. Sharp, op. cit., p2.

Essentially, the 1992 Agreement established a procedure for the parties to work cooperatively to secure compliance by Defendants with the remaining issues in the case, *e.g.*, individualized treatment, protection of patient rights, informed consent by patients to medication, proper medical treatment.

Significantly, and most importantly, this Agreement outlined an objective system for measuring compliance. *See* Monitor's Summary Report filed October 7, 1997, at 1–4. This evaluation system—Quality System Oversight (QSO)—was developed by Defendants in negotiations with Plaintiffs and the Monitor and is now nationally recognized as a method of measuring performance. Summary Report at 9.

According to the Monitor's Summary Report, all eight state hospitals are now in compliance with the 1992 Agreement. Seven of the hospitals have previously been dismissed from the Court's jurisdiction. The Monitor now recommends dismissal of the remaining hospital, Wichita Falls State Hospital. *See* Recommendation 37, filed September 25, 1997. The Court has reviewed the Recommendation and concludes that it should be granted.

This lawsuit has measurably improved the living conditions and treatment of patients in state hospitals. The violations alleged in 1974 have been cured. Unsafe physical facilities have been made safe. Stringent regulation of psychotropic medication of patients and informed consent by patients to medication are now standard policy in the hospitals. Patients' rights are established. The hospitals have more and better trained staff. The quality of psychiatric and medical treatment has greatly improved. There is increased emphasis on the importance of adequate care in the community for those discharged from the state hospitals. Provisions for placement of those who are both mentally retarded and mentally ill are now in effect.

The Court commends the constructive contributions of the current leadership of TXMHMR and its Board. The Court also commends the Texas Legislature for providing the funding necessary to accomplish the requirements of this suit. If such legislative support continues, maintaining the high standards now in place should henceforth be primarily a matter of good management and effective performance.

Of course, this case has not solved all of the problems of state and community care for the mentally ill. Much remains to be done in coordinating and financing care for those who return to the community from state hospitals. The necessity for sufficient funding by the Legislature will continue. More public awareness is needed regarding mental illness and the misery of those who are afflicted with it.[22]

---

22. R.A.J. v. Gilbert, Memorandum Opinion and Order, October 1997.

Appendix I: Appropriations TXMHMR

	1980	1981	1982	1983	1984	1985	1986	1987	
Central Office	359,202	374,524	641,033	674,010	822,502	828,886	530,975	530,975	
State Hospitals	124,068,875	128,321,690	156,367,165	167,394,174	174,476,071	176,601,803	177,080,299	174,506,899	
Contracted Community Services	46,829,898	48,570,141	58,102,388	61,407,904	83,872,982	84,856,544	91,095,521	91,095,521	
Staff to Patient Ratio	0	0	0	0	0	0	20,048,510	20,048,510	
Mental Health Construction	3,756,329	0	34,928,349	0	7,000,000	0	0	0	
OTHER	0	0	0	0	0	0	6,000,000	14,160,070	
Sub-Total	175,014,304	177,266,355	250,038,935	229,476,088	266,171,555	263,510,576	294,755,305	300,341,975	
Grand Total	393,329,990	392,818,644	525,985,533	510,358,217	589,129,351	582,370,424	620,174,527	618,630,159	

	1988	1989	1990	1991	1992	1993	1994	1995	Diff
Central Office	1,030,293	1,030,293	1,743,889	1,743,889	2,078,366	2,081,226	12,650,110	7,902,426	↑ 209%
State Hospitals	176,391,437	172,597,702	197,959,092	204,186,979	238,868,131	240,678,615	229,094,888	230,467,057	↑ 85%
Contracted Community Services	90,359,323	99,939,037	121,928,475	131,407,456	161,540,236	173,326,368	244,321,724	252,578,028	↑ 439%
Staff to Patient Ratio	14,896,787	18,265,738	0	0	0	0	0	0	
Mental Health Construction	27,623,216	5,731,430	62,203,445	300,352	63,397,093	5,002,504	8,373,400	0	
OTHER	18,198,382	18,198,382	19,103,486	19,103,486	19,103,486	19,103,486	28,360,553	28,630,553	
Sub-Total	328,499,438	315,762,582	402,938,387	356,742,162	484,987,312	440,192,199	522,800,675	519,308,064	↑ 196%
Grand Total	731,016,669	691,723,065	828,452,202	865,874,171	1,050,260,851	1,064,778,405	1,123,559,360	1,097,639,978	↑ 179%

Appendix II: Roles of the Actors in a Class Action Institutional Reform Lawsuit

The Court Adjudication Through:

- Hearings
- Court Orders
- Rulings
- Sanctions

Plaintiff's Attorneys:

- Advocate for clients (Expansion of scope of suit)
- Negotiate
- Litigate

Defendants

Agency

- Implement Requirements of Settlement Agreement
- Seek funding
- Represent Agency's Position Concerning Compliance

Attorneys

- Advocate for clients (Constriction of scope of suit)
- Negotiate
- Litigate

Monitoring Mechanism
Special Master, Court Monitor, Review Panel

- Advocate for Compliance with Consent Decree
- Monitor Compliance
- Present findings to Court
- Make recommendations to Court to support and advance compliance efforts
- Mediate between Parties
- Negotiate with Parties

Appendix III: The Life of a Class Action Institutional Reform Lawsuit

THE ACTORS

The Court	■
The Agency	▲
Plaintiffs Attorneys	□
Defendants Attorneys	▮
Court Monitor	○

■ →
Court Approves Settlement Agreement

▲ →
Agency Implements

○ →
Monitor Presents Findings

□▮ →
Contests Findings

■ →
Hold Compliance Hearing, Issue Findings and Sanctions

▲ →
Develops Corrective Actions and Further Implements

○ →
Monitor

□▮ →
Contests

□▮○ →
Negotiates Corrective Actions

▲ →
Implements

○ →
Monitor Recognizes Compliance

■ →
Court Dismisses Case

Chapter 11

Quality System Oversight

David Axelrad

The history of the R.A.J. lawsuit, the conflict between the parties over what constituted compliance with various requirements, and the resolution of this conflict through the development of a continuous quality improvement process have been described in previous chapters. This chapter will address the scope and history of Quality Assurance in the United States which has lead to the development of a Continuous Quality Improvement System utilized in state psychiatric hospitals of the Texas Department of Mental Health and Mental Retardation (TXMHMR). This Continuous Quality Improvement System is called Quality System Oversight (QSO). This chapter will provide a description of the clinical instruments utilized in QSO.

The foundation for Quality Assurance is both the generic definition of quality assessment coupled with basic principles of quality assurance. Quality assessment is defined as the measurement of the level of quality at some point in time with no specific effort to change or improve the level of care.[1] Utilizing basic mechanisms of Quality Assurance, one may establish the following principles that should be met in a Quality Assurance System:

Articulate a usable definition of quality

Establish mechanisms to develop professionally accepted standards

Create systems to collect and analyze relevant data

Disseminate findings

Implement and follow up corrective action

Avedis Donabedian, one of the fathers of quality assurance and quality assessment in medicine, has established that the epidemiology of quality must involve two more important elements:

---

1. Brook, R.H., Williams, K.N., Avery, A.D. Quality Assurance Today and Tomorrow: Forecast for the Future. Annals of Internal Medicine 85. (December 1976):809–817.

1. The study of distribution of quality at any given time

2. The study of its distribution through time

Donabedian has further elaborated the epidemiology and ecology of quality assurance with a definition of it's ecology.[2] One finds this description of epidemiology and ecology of assurance in Appendix 1. Upon review of Appendix 1, one finds that the epidemiology and ecology of quality requires the development of specific criteria to be utilized as the basic unit of data in the Quality Assessment and Quality Assurance process.

Quality Assurance mechanisms involve the development of criteria that are assessed through quality assessment mechanisms. The criteria in medicine would include structural criteria, process criteria, and outcome criteria. In addition, a fourth criteria has recently been developed which would include patient satisfaction with care.

Criteria in Quality Assurance do include both implicit and explicit criteria. Implicit criteria would include criteria that do not have a formal or written structure. The criteria are generally internalized expectations of an expert practitioner. Explicit criteria would be criteria with a well developed structure, allowing little or no room for individual judgment.[3]

The California Hospital Association and California Medical Association have developed a guide for criteria formation called RUMBA. Rumba stands for the following elements: R—relevant, U—understandable, M—measurable, B—behavioral, and A—achievable.[4]

Lastly, assessing the quality of care would include the need to define both the efficacy and effectiveness of care. Efficacy would reflect level of benefit expected when services are applied under ideal conditions. Effectiveness would concern the level of benefit when services are rendered under ordinary conditions by an average practitioner for typical patients.[5]

---

2. Donabedian, A. The epidemiology of quality. Inquiry. 1985;22:282–292.

3. Donabedian, A. Criteria and Standards for Quality Assessment and Monitoring. Quality Review Bulletin. 1986;12:99–108.

4. California Medical Association/California Hospital Association. Quality of Patient Care Workshop Manual. Los Angeles:CMA/CHA, 1975.

5. Lohr, K.N. Outcome Measurement: Concept and Questions. Inquiry. 1988;25:37–50.

Over the course of the development of quality assurance in medicine, one has found that there have been two basic quality assurance methods that have been developed. The first method is inspection to improve quality. The second method is continuous quality improvement. In order to understand the evolution of quality assurance into continuous quality improvement, it would be helpful to review the history of the development of quality assessment in medicine.

Upon review of the history of quality assessment and quality assurance in medicine, one finds that its history begins with the codes of physician behavior that are found in archaic sources including the codes that flow from both the Greek and the Judeo-Christian periods. These codes establish rules of conduct in ethical principles which guide the behavior of physicians and other healers.

In medicine, the association of medical superintendents established the first American standards for psychiatry in 1851. These standards were further adopted by the American Psychiatric Association in 1889.

In 1908, the American Medical Association adopted the Carnegie Foundation Flexner Report which further defined quality in medicine. A landmark study published by the American College of Surgeons lead to the hospitalization standard program of the American College of Surgeons in 1917 and 1918.[6] The Joint Commission on Accreditation of Hospitals (JCAH) developed further standards in 1951 which were followed by standards embodied in the Medicare/Medicaid Federal legislation in 1965. This lead to an expansion of the role of the federal government in health care regulations through the adoption of Public Law 92-603 establishing PSRO's in 1972.

In 1981, JCAH adopted a new QA standard titled Quality Assessment Standard which involved a single audit system to monitor clinical practice. This led ultimately to the development of a continuous quality improvement and total quality management system for hospital medicine in the United States by the Joint Commission of Accreditation of Health Care Organizations (JCAHO, formally JCAH). This lead further to federal development of standards through the Health

---

6. Roberts, J.S., Coale, J.G., Redman, R.R. A History of the Joint Commission on Accreditation of Hospitals. Journal of the American Medical Association. 8/21/76;258:936–940.

Care and Quality Improvement Initiative adopted by the Health Care Financing Administration. All of this history parallels the continuing evolution of continuous quality improvement, initially in industry and extending into health care and medicine.

Continuous quality improvement is a system of quality assurance based upon quality management methods which are statistically oriented and data intensive. Continuous Quality Improvement is a model that focuses on improving the process of producing typical care rather than using inspection to correct unusual areas. Total Quality Management and Continuous Quality Improvement involve quality planning, quality control, and quality improvement.[7] System improvement and continuous quality requires: a diagnostic phase — understanding the current system and appreciation of major factors involved in the diagnostic phase; a remedial phase — analysis of data relevant to criteria or standards, utilizing statistical processes; and an action or implementation phase — analysis of the data which leads to changes improving the system.

A review of the CQI System in state psychiatric hospitals of the Texas Department of Mental Health and Mental Retardation (TXMHMR), reveals this process of diagnosis, analysis, and actions. The five clinical instruments are the source of the data for this three step process. Implementation of QSO has resulted in substantial improvement in the quality of care as defined by the state psychiatric hospitals.

According to the theory of Total Quality Management and Continuous Quality Improvement (CQI), processes of service and production yield information may be analyzed statistically for the purposes of improving the quality of the service or product. As Burwick stated in his seminal article, Continuous Quality Improvement in Health Care, one may construct a Continuous Quality Improvement system in a health care setting with important steps in the construction process. The five steps are as follows: problem identification, targeting the assessment, measuring process and outcome of care, establishing criteria and standards for quality of care, and development of reliable and valid instruments to assess quality of care.[8] His fifth step of

---

7. Kritchevsky, S.B., Simmons, B.P. Continuous quality improvement; concepts and applications for physician care. JAMA. 1991;266:1817–1823.

8. Berwick, D.M., Continuous Improvement as an Ideal in Health Care. N Eng J Med. 1989;320:53–56.

Quality System Oversight   221

construction provides a starting point for the discussion of the instruments utilized in the Quality System Oversight Program (QSO) of the Texas Department of Mental Health and Mental Retardation (TXMHMR)—"Fifth, modern technical, theoretically grounded tools for improving processes must be put to use in health care settings.... Processes that can be improved by means of systematic techniques abound in medicine."

The development of the five clinical instruments in QSO are examples of Burwick's fifth step in the construction of CQI methodology for psychiatry. CQI requires that quality be assessed and defined in terms of specific measurable attributes or criteria (8). The most challenging aspect of the development of the measurement criteria involved asking the right questions and "deciding what to measure and how it should be measured."[9] The development of these instruments required extensive research of aspects of psychiatric and behavioral health care which influence quality. The instruments are consensual agreements between the program staff representing the parties and advocacy groups about the most seminal criteria for each issue. These instruments were developed and bench-marked in a number of field trials in hospitals selected for high quality of service.

These five clinical instruments are applied to a sample of charts on a monthly basis in the state psychiatric hospitals of TXMHMR (Appendix 2). QSO is a philosophy of CQI which incorporates the hospital's mission of quality service at all levels. The instrument's compliance targets must be met to demonstrate that the monitored activity is of acceptable quality. As discussed in chapter 4, the CQI system includes external review by a team of QSO consultants appointed by TXMHMR and a team of consultants appointed by the R.A.J. Court Monitor. The external QSO and R.A.J. teams undertake reviews of a matched sample of the charts which have been previously reviewed by the hospital's QSO team. These follow up reviews occur on a twice a year basis. These reviews are meant to validate the QSO activity in each state psychiatric hospital. In applying the instruments to this matched sample of charts, validity of the process is defined by an acceptable range of agreement (range less than 8.5%) between the hospital's QSO teams and the QSO-R.A.J. teams of TXMHMR. This range of agreement must be satisfied in order for the QSO activity at

---

9. Ibid.

the hospital to be validated. The state psychiatric hospital must meet the performance target and the range of agreement with the QSO-R.A.J. teams over time, as defined by the settlement agreement, in order for the hospital to be removed from the active QSO-R.A.J. monitoring by the federal court. It is important to clarify that the QSO process that has been developed in TXMHMR will be a continuing process long after the settlement agreement has been satisfied and the court has dismissed the lawsuit. Each instrument has both a compliance target and a matched sample range of agreement between the hospital's QSO team and the QSO-R.A.J. team.

The five clinical monitoring instruments in QSO are:

1. The Individualized Treatment Monitoring Instrument

2. The Medication Monitoring Instrument

3. The Medical Treatment Monitoring Instrument

4. The Consent to Psychoactive Medication Monitoring Instrument

5. The Special Procedure Monitoring Instrument

The monitoring instruments are composed of measurable criteria which define the quality of the process monitored by the instrument. Each of the instruments are applied to a patient's chart in a structured review. Each instrument includes a scoring guide which provides specific information and instructions concerning the scoring of each of the criteria of the instrument. The criteria in each instrument may be answered either yes or no, depending upon whether or not the criteria is satisfied pursuant to instructions in the scoring guide. The instrument provides important data which is subsequently analyzed utilizing tools of CQI analysis — i.e., pareto charting, fish-bone diagrams, cause and effect diagrams. This CQI review is an analysis of the system of care as defined in each of the instruments.

All of the instruments are applied to a sample of patients each month in each state psychiatric hospital. The sample is randomly collected and provides an opportunity to address system quality. Upon appropriate analysis of the data derived from this monitoring instrument, one may then determine areas needed for improvement. As previously addressed, all of the instruments are applied to a matched sample of charts in each state hospital twice a year by the QSO-R.A.J. team. Following the removal of the hospital from the active phase of QSO-R.A.J. monitoring, the QSO team continues to validate the process twice a year. Appropriate CQI methodology is involved in the application of the instruments.

The Individualized Treatment Planning Instrument identifies specific process steps which need to be done well in order for adequate treatment to occur. The objective of the instrument is to evaluate the quality of individualized treatment during the previous 120 day period of time. This instrument illustrates the important role of biopsychosocial assessment and formulation in both the diagnosis and treatment of patients in mental health systems.

The compliance target for this instrument is 80%. This means that at least 80% of the twenty-one criteria contained in this instrument should be affirmatively satisfied in order for the chart to meet the acceptable compliance target. The acceptable range between the hospital's application of this instrument and the QSO-R.A.J. application of a matched sample is 8.5%. If the range of variability is less than 8.5% during a specific site review, the QSO system in the hospital has been validated in that site review. The meeting of a percentage score of performance within the range of agreement signifies that the hospital is both performing at a desired level of performance and scoring the instrument within an acceptable level of agreement or calibration within a monitoring authority. The hospital and the monitoring authority are basically using the same yard stick.

Upon reviewing the components of this monitoring instrument one may note that the instrument utilizes the biopsychosocial model which includes both a systemic and multi-dimensional approach to diagnosis and treatment of psychiatric patients. It is based upon important hypothesis as defined by Sperry, Gudeman, Blackwell, and Faulkner in the text, Psychiatric Case Formulations.[10] All of the important components of individualized treatment are addressed in the instrument. These components include biopsychosocial assessment in terms of biological, psychological, and social considerations, the DSM-III-R diagnosis in Axis I, II and III, clinical formulation which yields a working understanding of the patient, based upon the biopsychosocial assessment, treatment planning, continual reassessment and reformulation of both the formulation and treatment plan,

---

10. Sperry, L, Gudeman, JE, Blackwell, B, Faulkner, LR: Psychiatric Case Formulations. American Psychiatric Press, 1992

changes in treatment when indicated, and discharge planning which assesses all of these areas.

These components of individualized treatment are assessed with twenty-one criteria which are quantifiable and define quality of individualized care. With application of this instrument, one may derive conclusions concerning whether or not the system is providing an acceptable quality of care of patients.

Criteria 1 through 3 involves biopsychosocial formulation in terms of biological, psychological, and social considerations. Criteria 4 through 6 requires that Axis I, II and III diagnoses are consistent with information found in the record. Criteria 7 requires a diagnostic summary and a clinical formulation, utilizing information obtained in the previous six criteria. The formulation includes integration of pertinent data of the assessments, an answer to the question—"how the patient became ill?"—a clinical basis for both the diagnosis and the description of the events which contribute to the acute illness requiring hospitalization. Treatment decisions should be documented with explicit rationale. Criteria 8 and 9 access treatment planning with addresses questions relating to diagnosis and treatment interventions, flowing from treatment objectives. It is important to note that these criteria address both the initial treatment plan and subsequent changes in the treatment plan with new information or changes in patient status. Criteria 10 through 16 involves the important elements of the treatment process—these criteria would include 20 hours of relevant scheduled programming, treatment relevant to the needs of the patient, documentation of patient participation in the formulation of the treatment plan, documentation by the physician of changes in patient status, documentation by the physician of the clinical rationale for treatment orders, progress notes from members of the treatment team reflecting the patient's target behavior as outlined in the treatment plan, and Criteria 16 treatment team progress notes reflecting staff interventions as outlined in the treatment plan. Criteria 17 through 21 involves critical elements of the treatment process. These would include continual assessment, reformulation and changes in treatment planning and discharge planning, continual assessment on the part of the treatment team, progress notes reflecting patient response to treatment, periodic team reviews and documentation of patient response to treatment, periodic reformulation, changes in treatment plan when indicated, documentation of patient's involvement in treatment plan changes, and discharge plans being appropriate to the patient's clinical needs.

The second clinical instrument, utilized in QSO, is the Medication Monitoring Instrument. The compliance target for this instrument is 85% in the first six months and 90% in subsequent time periods. The acceptable range of agreement between the hospital staff and the QSO-R.A.J. team should be less than 8.5%. The eight criteria of this instrument assess medication monitoring and the clinical rationale for both initiating and continuing psychiatric medications, and the effects of medication including the appropriate utilization of an AIMS Instrument and appropriate follow up of positive AIMS Scores. The first two criteria of this instrument access documentation of the clinical rationale for both initiating and continuing psychoactive medications. The third criteria addresses whether or not the physician has adequately noted both positive and negative responses to the medication prescribed for the patient. The fourth criteria assesses the clinical rationale for polypharmacy. Criteria five through eight refers to assessment of involuntary movements caused by psychoactive medications (AIMS).

A third clinical instrument is the Medical Treatment Monitoring Instrument. The objective of this instrument is to review and evaluate medical treatment provided to the patient during the previous twelve months. The compliance target for the Medical Treatment Monitoring Instrument is 80%. The acceptable range between the hospital staff and the QSO-R.A.J. team should be less than 8.5%. This instrument includes eighteen criteria. The Medical Treatment Monitoring Instrument measures the proper examination of the patient, assessment and evaluation of the patient to review medical/physical and history information, timely and appropriate reports, lab work, screenings, and consultations when indicated and of identified and reported injuries, illness, public health problems, and dental problems. This instrument was developed by and is scored by QSO/R.A.J. consultant internists.

The next clinical instrument in the QSO process is the Consent to Treatment with Psychoactive Medications Monitoring Instrument. The compliance target for this instrument is 85% in the first six months and 90% in subsequent months. The acceptable range of agreement between the hospital staff and the QSO-R.A.J. should be less than 8.5%. This monitoring instrument includes sixteen criteria.

This instrument measures the TXMHMR policy relating to consent to treatment with psychoactive medication. It is in direct response to needs for protection of the patient's rights for Informed Consent. The instrument measures the process of Informed Consent from competent patients or guardians, appropriate dates and signatures of participants involved in the consent process, assessment of the treatment alliance between the physician and the patient, documentation of administration of medications without consent during an emergency, and adequate explanation of the purpose, effects, side-effects, and alternatives to psychoactive medications. These criteria measure a reasonable process of obtaining informed consent. The following criteria measure the specific legal steps in Texas law for giving medications after a patient has refused the medication. These criteria include documentation of medication refusal, documentation of determination that the patient does not have the capacity to give consent, petition to the court when the patient appears to lack competence to give a consent, and documentation of 90 day medication reviews and renewal of consents. The Consent to Treatment with Psychoactive Medication Instrument also measures documentation of changes in medications within the same chemical class, documentation of changes in significant doses or in route or form of administration, and documentation of rationale for court-ordered medications. The application of this Instrument provides adequate assurance of the patient's rights to Informed Consent.

The last clinical monitoring instrument is the Special Treatment Procedure Monitoring Instrument. The objective of this instrument is to review the basis of evaluating the facility performance regarding departmental rules for providing restraint, seclusion, ECT, or aversive therapies. The time frame is the most recent 90 day period of the patient's hospitalization. The target compliance of this instrument is 85% in the first six months, and 90% in subsequent time periods. The acceptable range of agreement between the application of this instrument by the hospital staff and the application of the instrument by the QSO-R.A.J. team every six months, should be less than 8.5%. This instrument includes seven criteria. The first two criteria relates to the clinical rationale for initiating and continuing restraint. Criteria three and four refer to the clinical rationale for initiating and continuing seclusion. Criteria five involves the documentation of clinical rationale for ECT, criteria six—the clinical rationale for adverse therapies, and criteria seven—the clinical rationale for other special treatment procedures as defined by the relevant sections of the Mental Health Code of the State of Texas.

In summary, these clinical instruments define quality of care in the treatment of psychiatric inpatients. Appropriate pareto charting and other CQI methods of data analysis provide opportunities to address areas of need for improvement in the system. As one addresses the remedial and implementation phases of CQI and QSO, one must acknowledge two important pioneers of total quality management. Deming developed, throughout his long and productive life, themes and tools for improving processes involving planning, measurement, statistical activities, analysis, and recommendations (action) for quality improvement.[11] The Shewhart cycle (PLAN-DO-CHECK-ACT CYCLE) is a generic cycle that has been incorporated in the QSO process.[12] This process of CQI Analysis has resulted in significant improvements in the state psychiatric hospitals in TXMHMR.

Ishikawa has emphasized the importance of developing techniques of process flow analysis, control charting, and cause and effect diagrams to identify opportunities for change.[13] Deming's contributions and Ishikawa's contributions have played a most important role in QSO experience in Texas.

For the purposes of demonstrating how QSO meets both Deming's and Ishikawa's definitions of Continuous Quality Improvement, I will review for you the results of the application of three clinical instruments in reviews in the state psychiatric hospitals in TXMHMR.

Upon analyzing the performance of a state psychiatric hospital on the Individual Treatment Monitoring Instrument during the course one of our QSO-CQI site reviews, the score on the QSO-R.A.J. applications Instrument was 69%. This score reflects that the Individualized Treatment Monitoring Instrument did not demonstrate acceptable quality as defined by the compliance target of 80%. The next step in the analysis is reflected in a pareto diagram (Appendix 3). This pareto diagram demonstrates the percentage of "no's" that are nega-

---

11. Deming, WE, Out of the Crisis. Cambridge, MA: Massachusetts Institute of Techology, Center for Advanced Engineering Study; 1986.

12. Shewart, WA, Out of the Crisis. New York, NY: Van Norstrand, Reinhold Co: 1931.

13. Ishikawa, K, (Ed): Guide to Quality Control, White Planes, House International Publications, 1986.

228   State Hospital Reform: Why Was It So Hard to Accomplish?

tive responses to the twenty-one criteria of the Individualized Treatment Instrument. One finds that criteria #19, which is the criteria that reflects changes in the treatment plan when indicated, was 14% of the "no" responses on this Monitoring Instrument. Criteria #7, which is the criteria that requires a clinical formulation and integration of information from assessments, accounted for 9.7% of the "no" responses. Upon further analysis of the pareto diagram, one notes that criteria #1, the criteria relating to biopsychosocial assessment of the patient in terms of biological considerations, accounted for 9.7% of the "no" responses. Criteria #8, the treatment planning criteria, accounted for 9% of the "no" responses. Criteria #4—Axis I diagnosis being consistent with information in the record—accounted for 9% of the "no" responses. These criteria form the heart and foundation of acute treatment of psychiatric patients. While this pareto diagram does not reflect the remaining individual criteria accounting for the percentage of "no's," criteria #2 and #3, reflecting biopsychosocial assessment in terms of both social and psychological considerations, also account for a significant percentage of the "no" responses.

This CQI analysis of this specific instrument is utilized for the purposes of making important recommendations and changes in the system in order to improve the quality of individualized treatment. The hospital utilizes this pareto analysis of the percentage of "no's" on the Individualized Treatment Instrument to refine individualized treatment in those areas that were identified as falling below standards of quality. An action plan is developed to correct these deficiencies, yielding improvement in quality of the system.

Another illustration of a pareto analysis of the Individualized Treatment Instrument may be found in Appendix 4, which identifies the percentage of "no's" on the Individualized Treatment Instrument during a QSO-R.A.J. site review. The diagram reflects the criteria 7, 19, 8, 4, and 1 accounted for a significant percentage of the "no" responses. These criteria reflect formulation, changes in treatment plan when indicated, treatment planning addressing important clinical issues, Axis I diagnosis being consistent with information being consistent with information in the record, and a biopsychosocial formulation in terms of biological considerations. On this particular site review, the QSO-R.A.J. score was 81%. This reflected compliance with the compliance target which defines quality for this instrument. Nevertheless, the hospital is provided an opportunity to improve the quality of its performance by addressing itself to those criteria contributing to a significant percentage of the "no" responses on this QSO review. An action plan is developed which provides opportunities of improvement in those areas identified with a significant percentage of no responses.

Upon review of Appendix 5, this bar graph demonstrates that a specific state hospital in TXMHMR has experienced substantial improvement in Individualized Treatment Monitoring from April 1993 to June 1994. Over that period of time, the hospital's performance improved from 76%, on the Individualized Treatment Instrument, to 87%. The June 1994 QSO review demonstrated that the hospital did achieve the target compliance defined for this instrument which was bench-marked against hospitals in this country selected for their high quality of service.

Appendix 6 reveals a pareto diagram concerning the Medication Monitoring Instrument which was applied to a sample of charts during a QSO site visit. Upon pareto analysis of the Medication Monitoring Instrument, one finds a criteria #3 and #6 accounted for 30% of the "no's" and 20% of the "no's," respectfully. Criteria #3 refers to whether or not the physician's progress notes document the patient's positive and/or negative response to psychopharmacological interventions. Criteria #6 refers to whether or not the patient has had an AIMS assessment every ninety days. Criteria #2, accounting for 18% of the "no's" on this instrument, is the criteria that includes whether or not the physician documents the rationale for continuing psychoactive medications. These three criteria accounted for 60% of the "no" responses on this particular QSO review involving this Instrument.

Following such a pareto analysis, the hospital would then institute an action plan that would address improvement of the hospital's performance as defined by the needs for documenting patients' positive and negative responses to pharmacological interventions and a system to improve the administration of the AIMS Instrument every ninety days. The third area of deficiency, relating to the needs to document the rationale for continuing psychoactive medications would also be addressed with a specific action plan.

On review of Appendix 7, one may note the QSO performance from April 1993 until June 1994 in a specific hospital in TXMHMR. Upon analysis of this slide, one finds that in April 1993, the hospital's performance on the Medication Monitoring Instrument was 81% —

below the target compliance for acceptable quality on this instrument. In a subsequent site review in June 1994, the hospital's performance on this instrument was 90%, reflecting a satisfactory performance and compliance with the target for this instrument. One would assume that the hospital did develop an action plan that accounted for the percentage of "no's" found in the April 1993 site audit. Such an action plan was successful in view of the fact that the systems' quality demonstrated highly significant improvement as a result of the QSO assessment in June 1994.

Lastly, one may refer to a pareto diagram reflecting the utilization of the Special Treatment Procedure (STP) Monitoring Instrument (Appendix 8). On a particular site review, criteria #1 accounted for 38% of the "no's" and criteria #2 for 25% of the "no's." These criteria relate to whether or not there is documented clinical rationale for initiating and continuing restraint procedures. During this particular review, it was clear that the hospital's performance fell below acceptable standards of care. The hospital takes this information and utilizes it on a monthly basis.

Appendix 9 reveals the hospital's performance on the STP Instrument utilizing such pareto analysis. By demonstrating a need to document the clinical rationale for initiating and continuing restraint procedures, one may find that over time, the hospital's performance substantially improves. In this specific hospital, the performance on this STP Instrument went from 60% to 90%. One may find that the hospital's performance with the STP Monitoring Instrument did achieve compliance over time reflected by the 90% target compliance in the June 1994 audit. An action plan was obviously developed by the hospital in April 1993 that did contribute to substantial improvement in the monitoring of special treatment procedures. This obviously has relevance for both quality as well as patient rights.

It is important to clarify that the clinical instruments do have significant relevance to patient rights issues. The history of the lawsuit obviously flowed from the determination by the court that certain rights to treatment and other considerations were being affected. Most specifically, the Consent to Psychoactive Medication Monitoring Instrument and the Special Procedure Monitoring Instrument have a direct interface with the rights and monitoring that is a part of the QSO process. Psychiatrists, mental health professionals, consumer representatives, and family members play an important role in the application of all these instruments. This system has resulted in substantial improvement in health care quality in the state psychiatric hospitals of the Texas Department of Mental Health and Mental Retardation. The role played by psychiatrists, other mental health professionals, consumers, and family members is critical to the process. One may refer to Appendix 10 which illustrates how the QSO system has improved the quality of clinical care in state psychiatric hospitals in TXMHMR.

QSO Clinical Instruments Criteria

Individualized Treatment:

1. Does the core biopsychosocial assessment of the patient provide a clinical understanding of the illness in terms of biological considerations?

2. Does the core biopsychosocial assessment of the patient provide a clinical understanding of the illness in terms of psychological considerations?

3. Does the core biopsychosocial assessment of the patient provide a clinical understanding of the illness in terms of social considerations?

4. Are the Axis I diagnoses consistent with information in the record?

5. Are the Axis II diagnoses consistent with information in the record?

6. Are the Axis III diagnoses consistent with information in the record?

7. Is there a clinical formulation which integrates information from the assessments into a working understanding of the patient?

8. Does the treatment plan address the important clinical issues through the formulation of relevant identified problems, goals and objectives?

9. Do the treatment plan interventions logically flow from relevant treatment plan objectives?

10. Are there 20 hours per week of relevant scheduled programming consisting of core programs and activities?

11. Are the treatment interventions present relevant to the needs of the patient?

12. Is there documentation of patient participation in the formulation of the treatment plan?

13. Does the treating physician adequately document changes in the patient's psychiatric condition/mental status?

14. Does the treating physician adequately document the clinical rationale for treatment orders?

15. Do progress notes from the treatment team members reflect the patient's target behavior outlined in the treatment plan?

16. Do progress notes from the treatment team members reflect staff interventions as outlined by the treatment plan?

17. Do progress notes from the treatment team members reflect the patient's response to treatment?

18. Is there evidence of periodic treatment reviews which document the patient's response to treatment?

19. Were changes made in the treatment plan when indicated?

20. Is there documentation of the patient's involvement in decisions related to treatment plan changes?

21. Are current discharge plans appropriate to the clinical needs of the patient?

Medical Treatment:

1. Was a complete medical history documented within 24 hours of admission?

2. Was a complete physical examination documented within 24 hours of admission?

3. Were routine admission lab tests completed and available in the record within 72 hours of admission?

4. Were other appropriate lab tests, specific to the patient's physical condition and/or medical history, completed and available in the record within 72 hours of admission?

5. Was required annual physical examination completed within one month of anniversary date?

Quality System Oversight   233

6. Was required annual medical history completed within one month of anniversary date?

7. Were annual laboratory tests completed and available in record within one month of anniversary date?

8. Are all unresolved diagnostic issues and medically identified problems further assessed with proper screening, diagnostic tests and treatment?

9. If screenings, diagnostic tests or consultations are recommended, are they obtained?

10. If screenings, diagnostic tests results or consultation findings include recommendations for treatment, is there documentation that the physician considered such recommendations?

11. Did appropriate treatment result from screenings, diagnostic tests/consultation recommendations?

12. Were all current relevant public health issues diagnosed via screenings, diagnostic tests and consultations?

13. Did all relevant public health issues identified and diagnosed receive proper treatment?

14. Are documented complaints of illness or injury followed up with an assessment by a physician or a licensed nurse?

15. If recommended by the nurse, was the patient seen by a physician in a timely manner?

16. Did the physician provide treatment as needed for complaints of illness or injury?

17. Is an initial dental exam documented in the record within 30 days of admission?

18. If the patient had an acute dental condition, was treatment provided?

Special Treatment Procedures:

1. If restraint is ordered, is there a documented clinical rationale for initiating the procedure?

2. If restraint is ordered, is there a documented clinical rationale for continuing the procedure?

3. If seclusion is ordered, is there a documented clinical rationale for initiating the procedure?

4. If seclusion is ordered, is there a documented clinical rationale for continuing the procedure?

5. If ECT is ordered, is there a documented clinical rationale?

6. If aversive therapies are ordered, is a there a documented clinical rationale?

7. If any other special treatment procedures are ordered, is there a documented clinical rationale?

Medication Monitoring:

1. Does physician documentation include a clinical rationale for initiating psychoactive medication?

2. Does physician documentation include rationale for continuing psychoactive medication?

3. Do physician progress notes document the patient's response (positive or negative) to psychopharmacological intervention?

4. If the patients is receiving more than one medication having very similar or identical mechanism of action (polypharmacy), is the clinical rationale documented by the treating physician or by a written report or consultation from a qualified physician? (Such consultation will include assessment of the patient and review of the record.)

5. Did the patient have a base AIMS assessment within 72 hours of admission?

6. If the patient is receiving neuroleptics, has an AIMS assessment been completed every 90 days?

7. If the patient has a positive AIMS score, is there documentation of appropriate clinical follow-up/response?

8. After performing an AIMS screening on the patient, in your clinical judgment were the results of the previous AIMS screening accurate?

Consent to Treatment with Psychoactive Medication:

1. Is consent form in record?

Quality System Oversight   235

2. Is consent form either signed by patient (or when appropriate the patient's legally authorized representative) or is there documentation of oral or manual communication, (e.g., American Sign Language) of consent?

3. Is consent form signed by person giving explanation?

4. If the consent form is signed by the PA, R.Ph., or RN/LVN, did the physician confirm the explanation with the patient or the patient's legally authorized representative within two working days?

5. Is there documentation that all required information was discussed with the patient (or when appropriate the patient's legally authorized representative) regarding the psychoactive medication to be administered?

6. If medication was changed to a different medication within the same TXMHMR medication group (class) is there a progress note documenting for each instance that all required information was discussed with the patient (or when appropriate the patient's legally authorized representative) regarding the new prescription?

7. If there is a change in form/route of administration of the medication within the same TXMHMR medication group (class) is there a progress note documenting for each instance that all required information was discussed with the patient (or when appropriate the patient's legally authorized representative) regarding the new prescription?

8. If there has been a significant change in medication dosage within the same TXMHMR medication group (class) is there a progress note documenting for each instance that all required information was discussed with the patient (or when appropriate the patient's legally authorized representative) regarding the new prescription?

9. If psychoactive medication was prescribed and administered without the patient's consent, is an emergency situation documented?

10. If the patient or the patient's legally authorized representative refused psychoactive medication and/or withdrew his/her consent,

is this documented in the progress notes and on the consent form (MHRS 9–7)?

11. Has consent for psychoactive medication been reviewed with the patient or when applicable the patient's legally authorized representative at least every 90 days?

12. If the patient or the patient's legally authorized representative refused psychoactive medication following the patient's commitment, is there evidence that medication was reduced and discontinued or discontinued?

13. If the patient refused psychoactive medication and withdrew his/her consent, did the physician petition the court for a hearing for an order to authorize the administration of psychoactive medication as documented in the patient record?

14. If the court ruled to authorize the administration of one or more classes (groups) of psychoactive medication(s), is the order present in the patient record?

15. If the patient appealed the court order authorizing the administration of psychoactive medication, was the outcome of the appeals process documented in the patient record?

16. If the patient was prescribed psychoactive medication via a court order, was the medication discontinued upon the expiration date of the commitment?

Appendix 1
Epidemiology & Ecology of QA

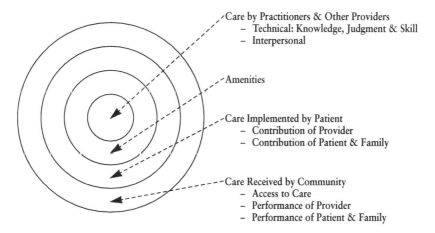

A. Donabedian
JAMA, 1988, 260:1734

Appendix 2

Five Clinical Monitoring Instruments: QSO

- Individualized Treatment Monitoring Instrument (R)
- Medication Monitoring 2-R Instrument
- Medical Treatment Monitoring Instrument (R)
- Consent to Psychoactive Medication Monitoring Instrument
- Special Treatment Procedure 2-R Monitoring Instrument

Look at Components of Individualized Treatment

- Biopsychosocial Assessment
  - Biological
  - Psychological
  - Social
- Diagnosis
  - Three Axis
- Clinical
  - Working understanding of the patient

Components of Individualized Treatment

- Treatment Planning
- Continual Reassessment & Reformulation
- Changes in Treatment
- Discharge Planning

Individualized Treatment Planning Instrument

Objective

Evaluate Quality of Individual Treatment During Period of 120 Days

Individualized Treatment Planning Instrument Includes 21 Criteria

1–3 Biopsychosocial Formulation

In terms of *biological*, *psychological*, and *social* considerations

4–6 Axis I, II, III Diagnosis

Consistent with information in record

7 Clinical Formulation Which Utilizes Information in 1–6 (Working Understanding of Patient)

Components of Formulation:

-> Integrate Pertinent Data of Assessment

-> Answer—How Did Patient Become Ill?

-> Clinical Basis for Diagnosis

-> Description of Events Leading to Acute Illness

-> Rationale for Treatment Decisions

8–9 Treatment Planning

-> Address Important Issues and Treatment Interventions (8)

-> Interventions Flow from Treatment Objectives (9)

10–16 Critical Elements of Process:

-> 20 Hours of Relevant Scheduled Programming (10)

-> Treatment Relevant to Need of Patient (11)

-> Document Patient Participation in Formulation of Treatment Plan (12)

-> MD Documents Changes in Patient Status (13)

-> MD Documents Clinical Rationale for Treatment Orders (14)

-> Treatment Team Progress Notes Reflect Patient's as Outlined by Treatment Plan (16)

17–21 Continual Assessment, Reformulation, Changes in Treatment and Discharge Planning

-> Treatment Team—Continual Assessment (17)

-> Progress Notes Reflect Patient Response to Treatment (17)

-> Periodic Team Reviews and Documents Patient Response to Treatment, Periodic Reformulation (18)

-> Changes in Treatment Plan when Indicated— Changes in Treatment (19)

>   -> Document Patient's Involvement in Treatment
>   Plan Changes (20)
>
>   -> Current Discharge Plans Appropriate to Patient
>   Clincial Needs (21)

Medication Monitoring Instrument

Objective:

> To Evaluate Quality of Medication Monitoring Being
> Provided to a Patient During the Most Recent 120 Day
> Period. Includes 8 Criteria

Medication Monitoring Instrument

Criteria 1–2

> Documentation of Clinical Rationale for Initiating and
> Continuing Psychoactive Medication

Criteria 3

> Positive and Negative Responses to Medication

Criteria 4

> Responses of Polypharmacy

Criteria 5–8

> Assessment of Involuntary Movements Caused by
> Psychoactive Medications (AIMS)

Medical Treatment Instrument (Measures)

- Proper Examination of Patient
- Assessment and Evaluation of Patient to Review
  Medical-Physical-History Information
- Timely and Appropriate Reports, Lab Work,
  Screenings and Consultations
- Treatment of Identified and Reported Injuries, Illnesses,
  Public Health Centers and Dental Care

Medical Treatment Monitoring Instrument (R)

Objective:

> To Review and Evaluate Medical Treatment Provided During Previous 12 Months. Instruments Include 18 Criteria

Medical Treatment Monitoring Instrument (R)

- Criteria 1–4 Apply to Patients Hospitalized for Less Than One Year

  - -> Complete Medical History Documented within 24 Hours of Admission (1)

  - -> Complete Physical Examination Documented within 24 Hours of Admission (2)

  - -> Routine Admission Lab Tests Completed and Available on the Record within 72 Hours of Admission (3)

  - -> Appropriate Lab Tests — Specific to Patient's Physical Admission (4)

- Criteria 5–7 Apply to Patients Hospitalized Over One Year

  - -> Required Annual Physical Examination Completed within One Month of Anniversary Date (5)

  - -> Required Annual Medical History Completed within One Month of Anniversary Date (6)

    Annual Laboratory Tests Completed and Available in Record within One Month of Anniversary Date (7)

- Criteria 8–18 Apply to All Patient Records. Instrument Applies to Medical and Psychiatric Care within One Year from Date of Review

  - -> Unresolved Diagnostic Issues and Medical Problems Further Assessed with Screenings, Diagnostic Tests, and Treatment (8)

  - -> If screenings, Diagnostic Tests or Consultations Are Recommended — Are They Obtained? (9)

-> If Screenings, Diagnostic Tests Results, or Consultations Findings Include Recommendations for Treatment—Documentation That Physician

-> Did Appropriate Treatment Result from Screenings, Diagnostic Tests—Consultation, Recommendations? (11)

-> Current Relevant Public Health Issues Diagnosed Via Screenings, Tests, and Consultations (12)

-> Relevant Public Health Issues Identified and= Diagnosed Followed by Proper Treatment

-> Documented Complaints of Illness or Injury Followed Up with Assessment by Physician or Licensed Nurse (14)

-> Patients Seen by Physician in a Timely Manner Following Recommendation by Nurse (15)

-> Physician Provides Treatment as Needed for Complaints of Illness or Injury (16)

-> Initial Dental Exam Documented in the Record within 30 Days of Admission (17)

-> If Patient Has Acute Dental Condition, with Treatment Provided (18)

Consent to Psychoactive Medication Instrument — 1 (Measures)

- Hospital's Attempt to Obtain Informed Consent from Competent Patients or Guardians

- Dates and Signatures of Participants

- Treatment Alliance Between Physician and Patient

- Documentation of Administration of Medication without Consent During Emergency

- Explanations of:
  - Purpose
  - Effects

- Side Effects
- Alternatives to psychoactive medications

Consent to Psychoactive Medication Instrument — 2 (Measures)

- Documentation of Medication Refusal
- Documentation of Determination that Patient Does Not Have Capacity
- Petition to Court and Cessation of Medications Prior to Determination of Court-Ordered Medications
- Documentation of 90-Day Medication(s) Reviews and Renewal

Consent to Psychoactive Medication Instrument — 3 (Measures)

- Documentation of Changes in Medications within Same Chemical Class
- Documentation of Changes in Significant Dosages or in Route/Form of Administration
- Documentation of Rationales for Court-Ordered Medications

Special Treatment Procedure Monitoring Instrument (2R)

Objective:

To Review Basis of Evaluating Facility Performance Regarding Department Rules for Provision of Special Treatment Procedure—During Most Recent 90 Day Period. Includes 7 Criteria.

Special Treatment Procedure Monitoring Instrument

Criteria 1–2

Restraint—Clinical Rationale for Initiating and Continuing Restraint

Criteria 3–4

Seclusion — Clinical Rationale for Initiating and Continuing Seclusion

Criteria 5

ECT — Document Clinical Rationale

Criteria 6

Aversive Therapy — Clinical Rationale

Criteria 7

Other STP — Clinical Rationale

Quality System Oversight 245

Appendix 3
ANALYZING PERFORMANCE
Pareto Diagram: Individualized Treatment

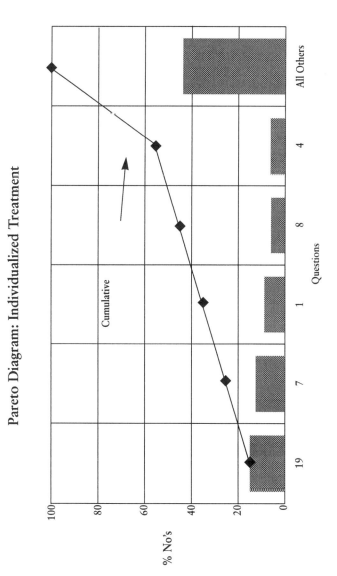

246   State Hospital Reform: Why Was It So Hard to Accomplish?

Appendix 4
ANALYZING PERFORMANCE
Pareto Diagram: Individualized Treatment

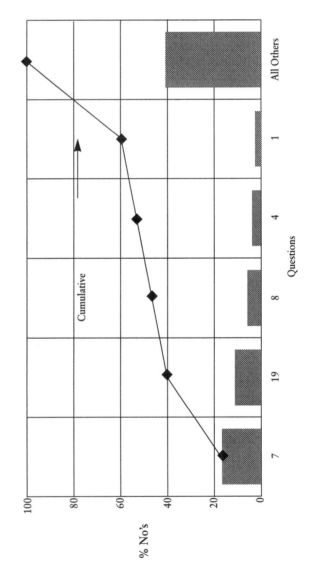

Quality System Oversight 247

Appendix 5
SEEING IMPROVEMENT
Individualized Psychiatric Treatment

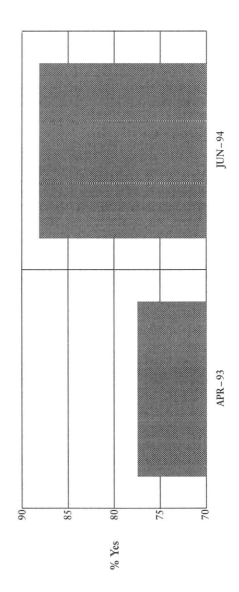

Appendix 6

ANALYZING PERFORMANCE

Pareto Diagram: Medication Monitoring

% No's

Cumulative

Questions: 3, 6, 2, 7, All Others

Quality System Oversight 249

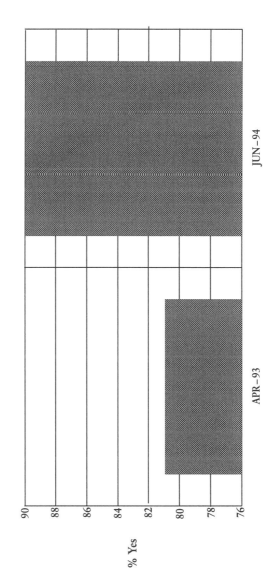

Appendix 7
SEEING IMPROVEMENT
Medication Monitoring

250 State Hospital Reform: Why Was It So Hard to Accomplish?

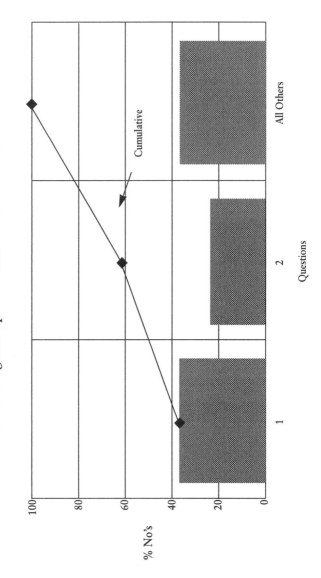

Quality System Oversight 251

Appendix 9
SEEING IMPROVEMENT
Special Treatment Procedures

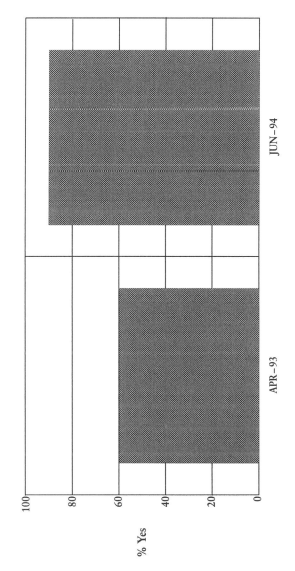

Chapter 12

The Consultant's Assessment of the Quality System Oversight Process

Art Farley, E.R. Hayes, Marty Lumpkin, Charles McDonald, Marilyn Clark, Lyn Henderson, Felicia Korman, Cynthia Patton Duran, William Smith, and Hazel Byers

The following vignettes represent the perspectives of a psychiatrist, an internist, several QSO team leaders, and several patient rights advocates who all participated in the reviews of the state hospitals after the 1992 Settlement Agreement:

THE QSO-R.A.J. PROCESS, AN ORDEAL OF CHANGE

Art Farley, M.D.

High quality medical-psychiatric diagnosis and treatment for every individual in the United States is a goal with which most agree. In Texas, a United States District Court mandated that quality medical-psychiatric care be provided for individuals without choice about the provision of their care. This Federal Court order presented a challenge to the Texas Department of Mental Health and Mental Retardation (TXMHMR) which has led a multifaceted effort toward meeting the court's mandate. The complexities involved in efforts to improve the quality of something as difficult as the provision of medical-psychiatric diagnosis and treatment in public facilities permeate the entire history of modern psychiatry. The efforts to assess quality care, to establish agreement on such an assessment, and to effect changes present enormous technical problems. This essay will be based upon a single consultant's personal experiences and observations of the QSO R.A.J. process.

A process which involves immense social, economic, and political pressures must be viewed from as many perspectives as possible and must have the capacity to survive the pressures upon it. Individuals without choice have little power and almost no voice when it comes to quality of care they receive. Outside forces were necessary in order to implement substantive changes in the public mental health system. Furthermore, the increased involvement of consumers in the health care delivery system in all sectors (public and private) has been a crucial ingredient and impetus for the process of change described in this book.

My initial experiences concerning the impact of litigation in the TXMHMR system occurred at the quarterly council meetings of the Texas Psychiatric Society in the mid 1980's. Gary Miller, M.D., representing TXMHMR as its Chief Executive Officer, attended these T.P.S. meetings on a regular basis and continued to attend into the 1990's. Based on Dr. Miller's reports on the status of the R.A.J. v. TXMHMR it appeared that the organizational position elaborated by TXMHMR was at base adversarial. As a Court Ordered Monitor was pushing for compliance with requirements of the lawsuit, this Monitor was being fought tooth and nail by the legal and leadership forces within the TXMHMR system. It appeared that non-compliance efforts must carry the day at all costs and that establishing compliance under the directives of the Federal Court and it's Monitor would undermine, if not destroy, the entire TXMHMR system. As a grim, disquieting, endless legal battle raged with both sides digging its heels deeply into the legal turf, there seemed to be no resolution in sight.

From one perspective, namely, the clinical practice of psychiatry and psychoanalysis, a substantial portion of the TXMHMR—R.A.J. situation resembled an extremely dysfunctional family system. One parent pitted against the other with everyone in the system suffering dreadful consequences, especially the children who basically had no choice in the situation. During this phase a satisfactory ending could not be envisioned because resolution seemed impossible. Consumers were essentially victims caught in this dysfunctional process with no end in sight.

At a grassroots level in Harris County, Texas, the local County Judge established a panel consisting of mental health providers and consumers—the Mental Health Needs Council of Harris County. This council researched the community's mental health needs and made recommendations to providers of psychiatric services especially for those individuals without choice who relied on public mental health care. As an example of the statewide dysfunction, there were several occasions when groups of discharged patients were simply dumped at the Greyhound Bus Terminal in Houston, Texas upon discharge from the TXMHMR hospital which served the Harris County catchment area. The patient received the harsh brunt of the legal conflict which seemed unresolvable over a protracted time frame. To an outside observer, it appeared that TXMHMR was going to battle against compliance with the R.A.J. Federal District Court decision. There would be continuing intractable divisive dysfunction in the public mental health delivery system with patient care and patient rights continuing to suffer.

In the fall of 1992, the central office of the Texas Society of Psychiatric Physicians (previously the Texas Psychiatric Society) contacted me and asked if I would serve on a panel of psychiatrists who would be willing to participate in a series of interviews conducted by the TXMHMR Quality System Oversight Office and R.A.J. Court Monitor. This was my first inkling that a change was underway which offered a window of opportunity for the potential resolution of the logjam described above.

A significant new component for change was the collaborative and interactive measures engaged in and undertaken by the TXMHMR-QSO Office and the R.A.J. Court Monitor. Although I did not participate in the initial efforts to create the instruments which would serve to collect data I was asked to review patient charts using these invaluable data collecting instruments which have been created to resolve definitions of compliance in the case. The collection of data in an organized fashion was a necessary first step toward useful collaboration between the providers of care (the hospitals) and the Monitors (QSO-R.A.J.). Everyone needed something that in some fashion resembled "the same page" in order to have the potential for useful collaboration.

There were many areas of overlap and interactions between all members of the QSO-R.A.J. teams involved in efforts to improve the quality of care in the TXMHMR system. I had been placed on the R.A.J. Court Monitor's team. Each member of the R.A.J. Court Monitor team had specific tasks and was paired with a member of the QSO team with the same tasks. Even though there was some diversity of training and experience amongst team members, there was an element of convergence which led to a somewhat surprising capacity to reach agreement on scores utilizing the clinical instruments previously determined. Substantial differences on clinical matters did surface between consultants; however, during the vigorous clinical discussions, utilizing the patients' charts as their data base, a score agreeable to both was generally found. When agreement could not be reached the matter was resolved by calculating the different scores into the total producing a high/low score or by an independent review of the differences by a separate set of reviewers. This systematic undertaking was called the "right answer process." From my perspective, this process has been one of the cornerstone elements which has led to the integration of continuous quality improvement into the TXMHMR system. It offers all participants, including the providers of care, an opportunity to present a more rational approach to monitoring treatment and to identify areas for improvement in the patients' care and management. When there is a rationale for treatment changes and it is explicated and understood, then, and only then, can systematic improvement of psychiatric services occur.

After multiple hospital clinical evaluations over a two year period, it became evident that some of the facilities were able to meet and achieve the quality improvements mandated by the Federal Court. Others seemed to be stymied. Efforts to assist those hospitals which were having problems were undertaken. Two person teams of consultants were sent to the hospitals which were having difficulty with compliance upon their request. I had the opportunity to participate in four team consultations to such facilities. I could never identify one common denominator as a single cause for all problems in the achievement of compliance. Hospitals in the system which were moving positively toward compliance did seem to have strong and deliberate clinical leadership which was clearly identified with the concept of a continuous quality improvement process. In the hospitals requesting help and consultation several factors seemed to impede the process even though the staff at these hospitals appeared to be dedicated to patient care and were working to improve.

Difficulty in achieving clinical compliance for some of the hospitals has been related to inconsistency of collaborative leadership at the highest clinical levels amongst all disciplines, e.g., medical, psychiatric, psychological, social work, and nursing. It was as if each discipline functioned separately with regularly occurring failures of communication. There was not patent organizational dysfunction and discord; it was sub rosa. In one hospital it was extremely clear that the data from the clinical psychiatric social worker was not integrated into the medical—psychiatric assessment and was therefore absent from the clinical interventions and treatment plans, thus inhibiting adequate quality care and appropriate discharge plans. Administrative changes or discharges were often not integrated into patient care strategies thereby creating dysfunction and disintegrating transfers of patients within the TXMHMR system. Nursing vital signs, although well documented, were not integrated into the overall medical—psychiatric assessment of a hypertensive psychotic individual's treatment plan, which led to a severe stroke with all the attendant sequelae. Team work and communication are crucial ingredients and yet hard to measure. When team communication is absent, the absence is felt and becomes glaringly apparent in retrospect. The effort at quality care improvement embodied in the QSO-R.A.J. process offers a striking opportunity to identify areas where improvements in care can be addressed in constructive ways. Each facility has its own history, ambiance, and means of addressing tasks. The QSO-R.A.J. process serves as a mode of approaching quality improvements which is flexible enough to address these differences.

The most unique personal experience in the QSO-R.A.J. effort involves my movement from the R.A.J. team component to the QSO team. I was asked to transfer from the Monitor's team to the QSO team at a time that the QSO team needed an additional psychiatrist. I feel that such an event reflects the constructive, non-adversarial component of the QSO-R.A.J. undertaking which was so adversarial and non-compliant at the outset. Ongoing potential for compliance and for continuous improvement in medical/psychiatric care has become integrated into the system. It would be naive to say that the forces which brought about the need for legal interventions will disappear.

E.R. Hayes, M.D., F.A.C.P.—Medical Care in a State Mental Hospital

This writer was a late comer to the R.A.J. monitoring the team. I joined the team in 1990. I was asked to measure the adequacy of the provision of medical care in the state hospitals which, although it had always been a requirement of the lawsuit, had not been measured previously. I joined the Court Monitor's team of psychiatrists and psychologists and did several reviews of medical care prior to the issuance of the Fourteenth Report to the Court. I submitted a report on medical care during that Report to the Court and then participated in the development of the medical instrument used in the QSO monitoring process. Once the 1992 Settlement Agreement was in place and the hospitals were monitored by the QSO instruments, I served as the internist on the Court Monitor's team and measured the hospitals while they remained in the active monitoring phase of the QSO process.

At the time that I began monitoring the hospitals in 1990 I had the impression that hospital staffs paid a great deal of attention to the economic utilization of medical resources. It rapidly became apparent that it was very easy to become focused on economics and neglect consideration of the quality of care given. This tendency became apparent to me during my first visit. We were reviewing the care that had been given one of the patients who had developed chest pain. The patient was in the age group in which most heart attacks occur. He had been put to bed, an electrocardiogram was done, and the patient was left to be observed until the following morning. No other medical tests were ordered. When I questioned why cardiac enzymes had not been ordered in series, the patient placed in a monitoring environment, and the other usual steps taken to rule in or out coronary artery disease and mild cardio-infarction, staff stated that if the EKG was not changed that other more elaborate studies were economically unwarranted for "this sort of patient." In response to further questioning several upper level staff openly stated that they questioned the value of this level of care for poor mentally ill patients. I took a firm stand that a two-tiered system of medical care would not be appropriate in a state system. I argued that the aim of medical care must be first class care for all patients regardless of their overall impairment brought on by their mental illness or their economic status. This attitude was not expressed again throughout the period of my monitoring. This concept that community standards of practice are expected for the patients in the hospitals became an important principle of the case.

As one studies the development and evolution of medical care in these hospitals it is helpful to understand that these institutions had involved from what were initially called asylums. These hospitals were places where impaired persons were taken care of for long periods of time. Little was offered in the way of treatment and rarely was a patient ever expected to be released from the institution. Their care was mostly custodial. The superintendent was usually a physician who was capable of caring for most of the physical ills of these patients. He may have been responsible for the medical care of 2,000 to 3,000 physically healthy patients.

The introduction of Chlorpromazine some fifty years ago caused a change in the type of care these psychiatric patients received. Many patients, under the effect of this medication, were able to live in open society. The face of psychiatry changed dramatically in these hospitals. The psychiatrist now became an active therapist. Psychoactive drugs became a hot item in the drug industry and new forms of these agents were being rapidly produced. The psychiatrists were hard driven to keep abreast of the rapid changes in their own rather new field. These physicians drifted farther and farther from the mode of medical therapy and were involved in their own psychopharmacology. This led to the overlooking or failing to care for non-psychiatric or medical illness in the patient. Many psychiatrists did not appear to be trained or equipped to manage the physical ills of their patients. This lack of training in many instances contributed to medical care which could not be regarded as meeting a community standard by the physicians trained in either family practice or internal medicine. A system of care that depended upon psychiatrists to deliver total health care produced inadequate treatment of physical ills.

Most hospitals did have one or two physicians who were trained in family practice or internal medicine who evaluated patients medically upon their admission. Patients then were placed under the care of their ward psychiatrist. In some instances recommendations by the examining physician were lost sight of and not implemented by this ward psychiatrist. This physician became involved in the psychiatric illness of the patient but focused his expertise in caring for what he considered the primary problem of the patient (the psychiatric condition). Medical illnesses therefore could remain untreated.

I brought these trends to the attention of the clinical directors of the hospitals during the first several years of our review of the medical treatment at the hospitals. Although the clinical directors generally used two methods to address these problems, for the most part, these organizational issues remained unresolved until later in the QSO process.

It is appropriate at this point to discuss our methods of evaluating the adequacy of medical care in the hospitals. Our evaluation was based upon the review of hospital clinical records. This may not be the best way to evaluate the quality of medical care but in our case it was the only way available to us that would allow the review of a large enough sample of patients to give us a reasonably fair judgment of the care the patients were receiving.

Our evaluation was based upon judgments of adequacy of the assessment, diagnosis, and treatment process of medical illness. We reviewed both routine admissions and annual assessment processes and then the diagnosis of acute problems. In our review we asked a series of questions which sought to evaluate the initial physical evaluation of the patient or the periodic reevaluation of the long term patient. We included in this appraisal the appropriate use of laboratory and x-ray procedures. We sought to ascertain if problems were properly and adequately addressed.

Our next area of concern was the detection and care of problems which might arise during the patient's hospitalization. I thought that this area was almost uniformly well handled. It gave me a good feeling that personnel were looking after their patients.

The next area of concern had to do with public health issues and their adaptation to the population of these hospitals. There were some problems usually revolving around attention to tuberculosis, the problems brought about by the HIV infection, and control of the hepatitis viruses.

During the active monitoring phase of the QSO process I reviewed charts and compared my answers with those of the internists on the QSO monitoring team. We usually had close agreement on our reading of hospital charts.

Early in the monitoring process it was apparent that problems lay in several separate areas. The first was the simple overlooking of physical problems in the entrance or interval evaluation of the patient and the second was a failure to take medical action once a problem was identified in the evaluation. In most instances the problems arose from either the wrong person being assigned the task of providing medical care or in a failure to follow through on the findings of the examining physician. In some instances it seemed that no-one ever noted the findings of the examiner and that many times the examiner seemed to feel no obligation to determine whether his findings and recommendations were being acted upon.

A third area in which many faults were found had to do with public health issues. There often was a lack of attention to tuberculosis screening, screening for HIV infection, and control of the hepatitis viruses. There was a general lack of preventive screening for people whose life style put them at risk of these illnesses.

It should be pointed out that at the beginning of this monitoring in 1992 that fewer than half of the hospitals had an adequate internist on their staff. It became the conviction of the QSO internists and myself that medical care should be provided by a separate medical service headed by a chief who is responsible to the clinical director for the entire institution. This chief of medical services should operate on the same level as a chief of psychiatric services. We began promoting this concept in our consultations to the clinical directors. Most clinical directors in the hospitals were receptive to this idea. The clinical directors during the last several years had been attempting to improve the quality of psychiatrists in the facilities and they now were faced with the need to recruit well trained internists to cover the medical needs of the rapidly changing populations in the institutions.

Each hospital began to make changes in the organization of their medical services but each hospital made these changes independently from each other. It is now worthwhile to describe the arrangement of services in some of the hospitals. One hospital had a well trained internist on the staff who had been made head of medical services in the institution. His presence as the chief of medical services demonstrated both the value of having a well trained internist active in the hospital and the value of a separate medical services.

At another hospital a well trained internist on the hospital staff had been assigned to work under the chief of the psychiatric services. Here, there was not the freedom of action in handling medical problems which could produce the high quality care that one might expect from this well trained internist. In another instance a well trained internist was assigned to the medical unit of the institution but was expected to perform the overall care of a large number of severely impaired psychiatric patients. This physician became so frustrated that his medical care suffered. It became apparent that this person was not the proper person to head the entire medical service. That position was filled by a medical specialist who did a good job as the administrator of the supportive medical services. The internist became a primary care provider; a role he performed well.

In another instance the supportive services were headed by an internist who was doing an unusually good job. However, he left the institution and a general surgeon took over the job as chief of medical services with the use of family practitioners and the use of consultants. The medical care continued at a high level.

There were hospitals that were slow to accept the idea of free standing medical services in a psychiatric institution. These were the last hospitals to raise the medical service to a compliance level.

At the same time that we suggested that the hospitals develop a separate medical service, we also suggested that the medical records be separated in such a way that medical physician notes could be separated from psychiatrist notes. In the past all notes, including psychiatrist notes, were in the progress report section of the chart. Physician notes were usually written in black ink and other notes were in other colors of ink. For a while this idea of separating physician notes from the rest of the progress notes was resisted but gradually each hospital made this shift. At this point medical notes are generally separated from the psychiatrist notes and both stand alone from the other progress notes. This facilitates the reading of the record.

I hope that these remarks will impart to the reader some impressions of the development of some operating principles which will lead us in our continuing struggle to improve the quality of medical care to psychiatrically impaired individuals. From the experiences of this monitoring project we may derive a few principles which can aid us in our constant drive to improve our art. It is important for there to be a definite supporting medical service which is separate and distinct from the psychiatric service. This will allow the widely divergent arts to be practiced at the same time on the same patients in the same institution. Properly trained staff must be available who are motivated to provide the highest quality of care to this impaired population. There must be flexibility in the organization of staff to permit for the maximum use of each staff person. This is an important reason for the separation of medical and psychiatric services. The fields are too large for the psychiatrist to be presently knowledgeable in medicine and for the internist to be knowledgeable in psychiatry. Much attention should be placed upon the prevention and early detection of public health problems.

Quality improvement can be attained. Our monitoring experience has demonstrated that. We do not work in a static situation but in a constantly changing one that demands our best efforts.

A View From A Crow's Nest: The QSO Team Leader

Marty Lumpkin, Ph.D., Charles McDonald, Ph.D., Marilyn Clark, M.A., Lyn Henderson, and Felicia Korman, M.S.W.

Since the beginning of the QSO project, the role of the QSO Team leader shifted. Looking backward, the phases of change appear as natural developmental sequences. But from the pastless perch of a pilot's seat, the same phases erupted rather than emerged as fragile products of multiple crosscurrents.

The QSO team leader role was created from the start of the QSO project. The purpose of the role was to posit a degree of leadership for the teams of consultants operating outside the boundaries of the TXMHMR Central Office and the R.A.J. court monitoring team. The role would ideally address fears that the QSO would be driven by a central bureaucracy pushing for court suit dismissal, or by a court monitoring group pushing for suit continuance. It was up to the QSO team leader to make the symbolic stand for continuous quality improvement as the driving force for the QSO process. Dismissal from the lawsuit, from this perspective, was but a by-product of the larger quality improvement initiative.

For the first year, the QSO leader role was largely symbolic. After the first year, the role gained in substance as leadership demands shifted toward it. Two forces slowed the development of the leadership function: the technical organization required for site visits and the need for on site negotiations on how to interpret various instrument scoring issues. The technical leadership of the QSO/R.A.J. teams came, at first, from the Central Office (TXMHMR) staff. The challenge to organize the efforts of over twelve consultants in order to get ample access to records for individual and "right answer" scoring, as well as to rapidly enter data to have an analysis completed by the last site visit day, was daunting and overwhelming. As technical bugs were worked out, leadership reins were gradually handed from technical problem solvers to QSO team leaders who could focus more on team process. The first year seemed to require more on site negotiated interpretations of scoring disagreements, in addition to the technical organization of the visits. The QSO team leader was not a formally empowered negotiator in the legal area, in contrast to the R.A.J./QSO Director and the R.A.J. Court Monitor. Looking back, the difficulty in clearly defining scoring criteria in initial stages, the lack of trust between TXMHMR and the R.A.J. team, and the uncertainty about where legal concerns split off from clinical/consumer scoring concerns all accounted for the heavy use of old leadership poles and the hesitant evolution of a new form of leadership "between" these poles. For the first year, the QSO team leader exercised symbolic leadership, i.e., representing the QSO team in meetings, and in process consultation. Without the symbolic or process functions, the team leader role would have slipped into an early obscurity.

After the first year or so, technical and legal issues solidified into more dependable boundaries, requiring less group energy to work through. The QSO team leader emerged as a key player as the need to manage group process grew in importance. Central Office staff receded into support roles. Troubled interfaces among QSO members, between QSO and R.A.J. members, between hospital staff and QSO/R.A.J. teams, or between Central Office and hospital staff were more and more managed by the QSO team leader and the Court Monitor. The chart scoring load of the QSO team leader was reduced to take on these process tasks. The development of comfort, trust, and a sense of shared values between QSO and R.A.J. allowed a parallel comfort on the part of R.A.J. consultants for the QSO team leader to be seen as a key facilitator and consultant to both groups. The role of process facilitator proved to be a critical one. A number of scoring issues were based on consultant interpretive judgments and the need for active, cooperative dialogues among team members. Without an atmosphere of mutual consultation across QSO, R.A.J., and hospital boundaries, the system would have easily vapor-locked into adversarial standoffs.

QSO team leaders and team members struggled with two dimensions of their roles in relation to the hospitals served—the role of auditor versus the role of consultant. As auditors, the QSO team's purpose was to score records and determine whether or not a hospital's scores could be verified as accurate and upheld to be in or out of compliance targets. As consultants, the QSO team's mission was to develop open dialogues with the hospitals' leaders in order to nurture continuous quality improvement perspectives and productive problem solving within this philosophy. The balance of these roles depended upon how the QSO visits were perceived by the hospitals. For the most part, these facilities, though usually cooperative, saw the QSO teams as people with sharp auditing pencils, not as consultants to welcome into the organization's own concerns or confidences. There were a few notable exceptions in facilities where CQI and the court suit were seamlessly sewn together. But the jury is still out. As more issues were dismissed from the court suit, QSO teams increasingly flew solo, without their R.A.J. counterparts. Most of the hospitals' tensions "to pass inspection" appear greater than the desire to move with QSO teams as collaborators toward a larger purpose—the full blossoming of CQI as the gold standard of quality improvement, and the need to use outside consultants beyond the lawsuit. From the perspective of QSO team leaders, this has been a constant vigil to look for opportunities for strengthening the role of consultants who bring not answers but outside-the-system viewpoints. Hindsight suggests that it is an almost impossible expectation to balance the roles of auditor and consultant when a lawsuit is in the foreground.

Casting a backward glance, in spite of hurdles and multiple frustrations, QSO team leaders still retain a perspective of passionate idealism about their roles. Their leader meetings remain focused on how to improve the effectiveness of site visits and how to offer their hospital "customers" systemic consultation. There is a real sense of pride binding this group of leaders. This pride is based on witnessing marked gains in the areas of treatment and consumer rights in most of the hospitals reviewed. And there is hope that the impassioned goal of continuous quality improvement will take on a life of its own apart from lawsuits and the tendency of bureaucracies to split off into competitive territories. The future of QSO is vision dependent: and that is a fragile source of power. If QSO and CQI blend in the facilities' own internal thrust toward quality enhancement, a critical transition will have been made beyond dependence on external forces provoking the move toward improvement At the time of this writing, the jury continues to deliberate.

Cynthia Patton Duran

As I drove to Dallas the morning of my interview with David Pharis and Doug Hancock I wondered where this opportunity would take me. It was an honor just to be interviewed. I had not slept much the night before because the excitement had made me anxious. I wanted to do well.

The trip from Marshall to Dallas took about three hours, so I had plenty of time to breed butterflies in my stomach. This was the first time for me to meet both of these men and I was nervous.

I had no trouble finding their office suite and they made me as comfortable as they could. The three of us talked about R.A.J. and patient rights for a while. We also talked of their roles in the lawsuit, then they focused on my background and what I could offer as a consultant.

My career as an advocate for psychiatric survivors was taking off well. I worked full time as an empowerment specialist for my local community MHMR, was serving on the Board of Directors for Texas Mental Health Consumers, and had just been appointed to the Texas Governor's Committee on People with Disabilities for the first of two terms.

I had always tried to make something positive out of any situation and see the brighter side of life. It was no different with my psychiatric disorder. I had been diagnosed in 1987 with manic-depression and spent two years battling the illness with numerous hospitalizations in the local crisis center. I entered a rehabilitation program in 1989 and I assured myself that I could overcome the stigma of mental illness and by doing so show others the way out.

I was thrilled when David Pharis contacted me and said he had chosen me for his team. Soon after, I received material in the mail that would be my bible for the next few years. I studied as much as I could but knew that I could not even imagine what to prepare for. Sure enough the pilot visit proved how ill prepared we all were. I was not ready for the chaos and tension that erupted between the teams and hospital staff which was to be the atmosphere for some time to come.

The first year was the hardest on everyone as we all struggled along. It took every bit of that year to gain confidence in my scoring. Being an advocate did not mean I was a rights expert. My background of expertise had been empowering consumers to advocate for better services. I was aware of patient rights mostly as a mental health consumer who had been hospitalized myself. I was not alone though in my frustration to do a good job for R.A.J. I remember Lyn Henderson, a Client Rights Officer who was a team member for QSO, experienced the same difficulties I had with scoring the instru-

The knowledge I now possess about the mental health field came mostly from working with the R.A.J. lawsuit. I usually read eight charts per visit and we visited each hospital twice a year.

At first it was hard to believe the rights violations that were handwritten in the charts, as if the writer was unaware of what was being revealed. Violations were a common occurrence.

Charts were often written in an unwittingly depreciating manner and all of the charts I read affected me in one way or another. For a couple of years I usually cried my way home after a visit. It was hard to read such harsh comments about my comrades in the hospital. Commonly I would read about a patient laughing to themselves for instance and the writer would treat it as an aberrant behavior. I thought there are times when I remember things that are funny and I chuckle to myself. I knew I could very well be reading my own chart. It frightened my sense of reality.

At all times when I read a violation I made sure I could back it up with written facts because there were often loopholes that many violations fell through and we could not score.

Almost half of the Patient Rights Instrument was taken up with questions pertaining to filling out one single form, the Patients' Explanation of Rights Information, which was given within twenty-four hours of admission and yearly. Many hours of debate and discussion was spent on the proper way to fill out this form. It was aggravating to me to see so much energy put into that when quite often I could only score multiple and more serious violations on one question that grouped them all together.

There were charts that had violations such as personal property taken away, monitored phone calls, to more serious ones such as an injury abuse case that was grossly mishandled.

The charts I read might contain one or all of these violations but could only be scored on one question in the instrument that asked if there were any violations. Filling out the Patients' explanation of Rights form, in my opinion, could have little impact on improving conditions for the patient.

It seemed to me that as soon as the hospital staff learned to initial the proper spaces the hospitals started coming into compliance with the lawsuit and closed the patient rights area quickly.

During the right answer process things could get rather volatile. Tempers flared and the arguments over the scores seemed to get personal. To change one's score meant defeat or insult to some. Some individuals would not change their scores no matter how obvious the facts were and others were enlightening to work with.

The conflicts encountered during the right answer process were carried into the group meeting where everyone became involved. We felt very rushed as there was not enough time for everyone to speak their piece and complaints were voiced if certain groups took up too much time in discussion.

I hated the position some professionals took about the value of advocates' opinions. There were definite lines drawn between some of us. We hashed out our differences and agreed to disagree on occasion. I felt I had to fight harder to get my points across because I did not have the credentials of a professional to back up what I was saying. My stance was driven by instinct and personal experience as a patient, which was unique and valuable to some.

Marty Lumpkin was a professional that I felt safe exploring this issue with. He had the gift of treating everyone equally. I went to him for a reality check about my paranoia and he confirmed that some people were just that way.

Without the support of David Pharis and the team he chose I doubt if I could have made it through this task. I remember telling David how insecure I was with my scoring and he readily assured me that I was as good as anyone.

I remember with pleasure the conversations I had with Dr. Raymond Leidig and Dr. Nina Muse. They answered my questions and fed my curiosity with honesty and open mindedness. They inspired me.

I relish the time I spent with Dr. David Bell. His humor kept me laughing when I sometimes felt like crying. He is a special individual that I will never forget.

Donna Cox and Dwight Spears gave me friendship. Many times they were sounding boards on how to handle difficult issues. Without them I would have walked around with my foot in my mouth most of the time.

As teams we had separate, though similar functions. Cindy Hopkins, from QSO, was my most difficult counterpart. Her intelligence and expertise on patient rights were unsurpassed by anyone. She knew the laws and codes like the back of her hand. Cindy told me of the hours and days she studied and she encouraged me to work harder.

Comparing the roles I played, one as R.A.J. consultant and one as psychiatric consumer, I cannot help but wonder, "Did we do anything but teach hospitals how to record charts without violations?" This jaded thought comes from my experiences with recent hospitalizations after the work we put into compliance monitoring.

I feel more stigma now with my mental illness than I did ten years ago when I was first diagnosed. In the state hospital where I was a patient intermittently from 1995 to 1997, I was abused and overmedicated. I also witnessed others treated the same way.

The last time I was hospitalized there was in February 1997. This particular hospital was among the first to be released from the lawsuit in the areas of patient rights and abuse and neglect.

During my stay I experienced an extreme attack that acted like a seizure. I was nonviolent and lying on the ground as it happened. Two aides roughly picked me up and carried me to the seclusion room on my ward without assessment of my condition.

They chose this time to take my jewelry. One male aide severely sprained and bruised my finger taking off a ring. A nurse shot me in the hip with a tranquilizer that I had stated on my chart that I could not take. Then they closed the door and locked it. I felt the stiffness of the Haldol take effect. I was alone and scared. I laid there feeling dehumanized and tried to collect myself.

I have been conditioned enough to know the quickest way out of a seclusion room is to become totally submissive. I cried. After what seemed like an eternity a staff person unlocked the door and my pulse quickened. Just because they opened the door did not mean I was going to get out. I had to pass the test.

The staff person talked to me in a parental tone of voice asking me if I was going to be "good." I had been in there for awhile and I desperately needed a cigarette. I still felt like my brain was in some type of seizure, plus the fog of the Haldol was disconnecting my senses.

I did not know what I had done wrong. I was frightened and felt ashamed for even being there. On several occasions I requested another doctor but was refused.

I felt I had no rights in there. The atmosphere was charged with constant tension. A young woman who was several months pregnant was incited to act out and repeatedly strapped down to her bed for hours. It was Bedlam.

This is a rather typical scene that I have witnessed in state, community, and private mental hospitals. It has happened to me and others many times. It is a common occurrence that nobody likes to talk about or publicize in our day and age but nonetheless it is my reality.

Hospital staff who work directly with the patients during most of their shift come from varied backgrounds with little psychological training or education. Some I have met had been employed in construction, truck driving, and restaurant jobs before going to work as a direct care staff for the hospital. These individuals got crash courses on how to manage aggressive behaviors with take downs and other physical interventions. This is usually a one or two day training class given by the hospital.

Oddly enough the hospital staff with the most education serves the least amount of time with the individual patient. There is very little one-on-one counseling as opposed to maintenance with tranquilizing medications.

I hope that since R.A.J. is settled maybe now the laws will not just be an experiment, they will be something concrete to enforce. I believe we still have a long way to go in mental health services but we all worked hard for R.A.J., the plaintiffs and team members alike, and I know it meant something for our future.

William Alexander Smith, Ph.D. — Consumer Rights Advocacy

My involvement in consumer rights for the mentally ill goes back several decades. Only recently, however, has it taken an active role predicated by my joining the Brazos Valley Alliance for the Mentally Ill (BVAMI) in 1991. This membership led to my joining the Quality System Oversight (QSO) team of TXMHMR in 1992.

The Consultant's Assessment   271

I report on my participation in the QSO process in a general sense to protect confidentiality, at monthly BVAMI meetings. This reporting has established credibility for the QSO work with this local advocacy group for the mentally ill.

Our four areas of expertise as QSO members involves patient rights, hospital unit rights review, patient abuse and neglect, and patient satisfaction surveys. I have received substantial satisfaction from my participation in this process. First is the sense of helping the mentally ill as evidenced by improving levels of hospital management and improved patient satisfaction with their hospitals. Second is the continuing improved response to change by hospital staffs. Attitudes are changing to where our visits are openly anticipated to help them improve patient care. In most instances hospitals are anxious to follow recommended changes.

Some adversarial relationships continue to exist but over time these are more positive. On occasions our work load is excessive causing scoring errors. This is being alleviated by increases in consumer rights advocates visiting each hospital. All in all this advocacy is a very positive and rewarding experience.

Hazel Byers

The following are bits and pieces of my recollection of the QSO/R.A.J. monitoring process:

The team members overall are an interesting, well selected group of people who make an effort to get along with each other. The few difficulties that I had in the beginning seem to be solved as the process of monitoring continued. In the beginning there seem to be more turfism; but as the process continued the reviewers became more accommodating.

In the beginning, the hospital staffs seemed apprehensive and angry over our presence. It seemed as if they believed we were out to get them. As time went on each hospital started expecting us and seem to look forward to our visits. Now, I am always greeted with a friendly smile and many staff know me by name.

It has been interesting to watch the improvements of patient care during this process. Taking our suggestions and recommendations, the staffs of the various hospitals seem excited to realize how well they work. To change their procedures is not only a lot of hard work but mind altering as well. I get the message that not only are the positive changes coming about to satisfy the lawsuit but staffs of the various hospital are on a trip they did not know existed or could exist some years ago before the process started.

A great deal of effort went into planning the instruments and procedures used by the reviewers. As time passed, we realized some of the questions or procedures needed to be changed. We needed to update our questions and become more efficient in order for all work to be correctly done in the time allowed. People worked willingly together to improve the work processes. It was exciting to be a part of this process. I appreciated being a part of the instrument revision meetings because the monitors became part of the process rather than being told what needs doing. There is much good information that the monitors are allowed to offer the process.

The right answer process in the active phase of monitoring was important because it fulfilled an educational function and because it improved the overall measurement. Two opinions were sometimes better than one.

The conferences with the staff in the beginning were difficult at best. However, as we each became more comfortable with each other, more and more good information was passed to the hospital staff. As the process took hold, the reviewers changed our schedule to include more staff people in our day by day work and in our summary sessions. I believe the staff appreciated being included in the summaries. They did not feel left out. Everything was up and above board.

It is exciting to return to the various hospitals to see our recommendations taking place—to see the improvements.

My biggest complaint is the poor handwriting on progress notes and doctor's orders as well as charts not always in proper order. People who chart need to write more clearly and precisely. Note taking as an art needs to be taught to the charting staff. There needs to be a more resume style of charting.

Chapter 13

The Legacy of R.A.J. from the Court's Perspective

Barefoot Sanders

Some may believe that the R.A.J. suit completely resolved all issues involving Texas' mental health hospitals for the future as well as the present; they would be incorrect. Some few may argue that the progress achieved by the litigation would have occurred without it; they, too, would be wrong. Some will say that a great deal was accomplished and the foundation laid for continuing progress; they would be right.

In hindsight, the R.A.J. case may fairly be considered as having gone through three stages—the initial and semi-dormant period, 1974–81; the contentious period, 1981–92, following the 1981 settlement; and the relatively harmonious final period, 1992–97, following the 1992 settlement.

The 1974–81 stage began with the filing of the case by the Legal Services Corporation in 1974 against eight Texas mental hospitals. Jurisdiction of the federal court was invoked based on alleged violations of federal constitutional rights. Violations of state statutes were also alleged. The specific federal constitutional violations included abuse of medications, unsafe physical conditions, unlawful restraints, and failure to protect patients' rights. The case was certified as a class action. In 1977 the United States Department of Justice entered its appearance as amicus curiae and for the next ten years played a major and constructive role in the litigation.[1]

The 1982–92 stage began with the Settlement Agreement reached by the parties and approved by the Court in 1981, and the appointment by the Court of a Review Panel in 1982 to assist the Court in

---

1. The Justice Department withdrew from the case in the late 1980's, stating that it was unable to support the position of the Court and the Monitor with respect to community aftercare.

monitoring and enforcing the terms of the Settlement.[2] For the next decade considerable progress was made toward meeting the requirements of the Settlement Agreement. Some issues were resolved and released from the Court's jurisdiction. Legislative funding for the hospitals—not generous but minimally adequate—increased. The Panel, and later Mr. Pharis, actively patrolled compliance with the Settlement and filed periodic reports and recommendations with the Court.

However, the Defendants often disagreed with those reports and recommendations. The disagreements usually revolved around interpretations of the Settlement. The disputes became more frequent. The attitude of the Commissioner of the Texas Department of Mental Health and Mental Retardation (TXMHMR) and his attorneys toward the litigation was increasingly negative. Resolution of the remaining issues in the case seemed remote. In October 1990 the Court named Mr. Edward Cloutman, a Dallas attorney experienced in institutional reform litigation, as lead attorney for Plaintiffs to assist the Legal Services' attorneys. In 1991 the Court directed counsel for the parties and the Monitor to confer and try to reach agreement on what actions had to be accomplished in order to fully resolve the remaining issues in the case. These discussions culminated in the 1992 Settlement.

The 1992–97 period was highlighted by the Court's approval of the 1992 Settlement, the principal feature of which was the establishment of Quality System Oversight (QSO) which provided relatively objective criteria to measure each hospital's progress in meeting and adhering to defined acceptable standards of care. New leadership at TXMHMR brought a more positive approach to the litigation. The teams which monitored hospitals for compliance with QSO, working with the Monitor, brought a professional point of view to their task. During the five-year period all eight hospitals were brought into compliance with QSO. In October 1997 the Court held an evidentiary hearing and determined that the unconstitutional treatment and conditions to which the case was directed had been remedied and that the hospitals now had the funds and effective management necessary for continued compliance with the 1992 Settlement. The Monitor,

---

2. Without objection the Court later replaced the Panel with Mr. David Pharis as R.A.J. Monitor. Mr. Pharis had been serving as Chair of the Panel.

Mr. Pharis, and the Plaintiffs supported dismissal of the case; TXMHMR officials in their testimony promised continued compliance. The Court therefore entered Judgment of Dismissal.

As has been noted, it may be argued by a few that the reforms made since R.A.J. was filed in 1974 would have been made without the litigation. History and experience do not support that view. In Texas and elsewhere such reforms seem always to require a judicial shove. Legislators and administrators are slow to act. Many legislators are not aware that constitutional violations exist until a lawsuit is filed. Patients in the hospitals have no political muscle. Administrators do not have funds to make improvements even if they wish to. And improvements cost money; absent strong leadership at the state level, increased state appropriations for mental hospitals do not bring public acclaim. R.A.J. focused the attention of state leadership and the public—and, importantly, brought the spotlight of media attention—to the conditions of the state hospitals and their patients.

Like similar lawsuits in other states, the R.A.J. litigation moved slowly. Legislators and state and local agencies have a visceral resistance to federal court "interference."[3] Tact and firmness by the Monitor (or similar official, e.g., Special Master) and the Court can mitigate but not completely alleviate this attitude. The attitudes of counsel for the parties are important, too. Lawyers are by nature and definition adversarial; indeed, that is what many clients expect. But in institutional reform settlements the adversary approach must be somewhat tempered for there to be progress.

During the 1981–92 period, in addition to constantly interpreting the 1981 Settlement, the Court was confronted with changes in case law. When R.A.J. was filed in 1974 it was generally accepted that the federal court, with clear jurisdiction of alleged violations of federal rights, also had pendent jurisdiction of violations of state law. Both federal and state violations were alleged by Plaintiffs in R.A.J. and the Court's jurisdiction to act in both areas was evidenced by the provisions of the 1981 Settlement. However, during the 1980's, the law as enunciated in court decisions began to change. The Supreme Court stated that a "federal court...must identify a [federal] constitutional

---

3. The Court's observations are based on experience with three institutional reform cases—R.A.J., Lelsz v. Kavanagh, (a sister case involving schools for the mentally retarded in Texas), and Tasby v. Hughey, the Dallas school desegregation case. Notably, all of these cases commenced in the early 1970's.

276 State Hospital Reform: Why Was It So Hard to Accomplish?

predicate for the imposition of any affirmative duty on a state." See Youngberg v. Romeo, 457 U.S. 307 at 319, n. 25 (1982). This was followed by Society for Good Will to Retarded Children v. Cuomo, 737 F.2d 1239, 249 (2nd Cir. 1984) holding that there is no federal constitutional right to community placement for the mentally retarded. In the same year, in a 5–4 opinion, the Supreme Court, citing the Eleventh Amendment, held that a federal court cannot enter judgment against state officials for violation of state law, the state in question (Pennsylvania) not having consented to federal jurisdiction. See Pennhurst State School, et al. v. Halderman, et al., 465 U.S. 89, 102, S.Ct. 900 (1984). Pennhurst was a contested case, not a settlement.

Of course, in R.A.J., Defendants had entered into the 1982 Settlement, thus (presumably) consenting to federal jurisdiction. But in Lelsz v. Kavanagh, 807 F.2d 1243, reh'g. en banc denied, 815 F.2d 1034, cert. dism'd., 483 U.S. 1057 (1987) the Fifth Circuit, in an 8–7 decision, held that

> ...mental patients have no federal right to a least restrictive living environment. Such a right is granted only by state law....the district court on remand may not enforce the consent decree in a way that requires the state to provide care to mental patients in a least restrictive environment.

This extended the Pennhurst restriction to consent decrees. That Lelsz involved the mentally retarded while R.A.J. concerns the state hospitals for mental health is a distinction without a difference.

This Court doubts that community aftercare can feasibly be considered separately from care in the state hospitals; indeed, both the 1981 and 1992 Settlements recognized the importance of an effective community care system. But the Lelsz holding has vitiated the authority of federal courts in community aftercare, at least in the Fifth Circuit.

Other negative developments in the law affecting federal institutional reform suits must be briefly mentioned. Beginning in the 1980's the Legal Services Corporation, which had often initiated such suits, was restricted by legislation and decreased appropriations in its ability to bring such suits. Private attorneys rarely have the resources or time to conduct such litigation. Institutional reform suits are now rare. It seems unlikely that such suits have faded because conditions in hospitals in every state have so improved that federal constitutional violations no longer exist.

Additionally, the current agitation for federal legislation to require constant review and justification for continuation of a federal consent decree must be noted. While the federal courts cannot be deprived of jurisdiction of federal constitutional violations, their reliance on settlements by way of consent decrees can be discouraged by legislative requirements for frequent hearings and review. The result may well be more trials and fewer settlements when and if institutional reform suits are brought in federal court. The result may also be that state courts will attract more institutional reform suits that previously have been brought in federal court.

The R.A.J. suit has brought benefits in addition to remedying unconstitutional treatment and conditions and the establishment of QSO. There is an increased public awareness of the mental hospitals and their patients. The legislature is more keenly attuned to the needs of the hospitals. The kind of legislative and administrative neglect which existed pre-R.A.J. is unlikely to recur soon. Of course, if appropriations lag or if QSO standards are relaxed or not enforced, the violations which R.A.J. remedied will haunt the state again.

It may legitimately be asked if the Court should have ordered continuing judicial supervision of the hospitals. However, permanent federal oversight is neither feasible nor desirable. The Court does not have the resources for such stewardship. With unconstitutional conditions largely cured, the operation of the hospitals had to be returned to the state as the governmental authority principally responsible for their funding and operation.

In sum, then, the legacy of R.A.J. is this: the purpose of R.A.J. was to improve the conditions and treatment of patients in Texas' mental hospitals. With perseverance by the Court and the Monitor and a constructive attitude by the Legislature and TXMHMR the purpose of the lawsuit was achieved.

Afterword

David Mechanic

This narrative of efforts to bring significant change in public mental hospitals in Texas over a 23-year period evokes many reactions and emotions. One can feel the anguish of persons with serious mental illness and their families confronting the unpredictability and uncertainty of their lives and marvel at their courage. One can sense the frustration of a court and its representatives in experiencing the difficulties of change and the intractability of legislatures and large public bureaucratic systems. One can sympathize with mental health workers and administrators struggling to carry on with very limited resources only to have their motives and humanity questioned and criticized. One can even empathize with the politicians fully aware of the inadequacy of the health safety net, knowing that if they raise taxes to repair it, voters will probably punish them.

A highly strained staff, caring for too many difficult and sometimes violent patients, may adopt practices that help control their fears and uncertainties but are dehumanizing to patients. A hospital administrator, struggling with limited resources and staff, may triage patients in ways that denies some a decent level of humane care. A court may impose requirements that give those having care responsibility too little flexibility to use their best professional judgment under difficult cost restraints. Most are decent people doing their jobs as best they can but sometimes without awareness of what they leave in their wake. In understanding their behaviors we need not condone them. Instead we have to design organizational strategies and approaches that make it more possible to offer a decent level of service. The Quality System Oversight eventually put in place in Texas public mental hospitals is one such example.

Personality and context played a role in this long and tortuous lawsuit. All of the mental health commissioners found the court's interventions constraining and counterproductive in some ways, but each responded differently making attempts at resolution more or less acrimonious. Lawyers representing each side, playing their usual advocacy roles, no doubt heightened the acrimony, but some were better able than others to rise above the adversarial battle and help define a common interest. Core to the process was trust, and the willingness of each of the involved participants to take the risks that trust required. But we miss the point if we simply focus on personalities and participants' chemistry with one another. What was often missing was adequate process for effective conflict resolution.

David Pharis estimates the cost of this lawsuit over 23 years at $7 million but this is a vast simplification not only of the financial costs but, more importantly, the social costs. How many thousands of hours were spent by administrators and professionals analyzing, strategizing, and deflecting some of the requirements being imposed? How does one measure the anger, frustration and humiliation of those who in trying to do their jobs are being vilified in the press? What costs for the system does diminished esteem and morale of thousands of mental health staff have, and what price do patients pay as a result? The cost-benefit calculations are difficult and solutions evasive. But there has to be a better way.

The State of Texas has a long history of neglecting its most disadvantaged citizens. For years it has ranked at the bottom among states in per capita expenditures for mental health, and it looks even worse when its income and wealth are taken into account. Yet it has often been the context for innovative practice and impressive leadership in mental health. I am an outsider to Texas, but have had some opportunity to observe mental health developments, first as a consultant for the Robert Wood Johnson Foundation Program for the Chronically Mentally Ill and site visitor to the Austin-Travis County Mental Health and Mental Retardation Center, and later as a member of the National Advisory Council of the Hogg Foundation for Mental Health during the period of their statewide commissions on the mental health of Texans. In these endeavors, I was repeatedly impressed by the talent, creativity, dedication, and good will of many family members, advocates, mental health professionals and administrators throughout the state. In reviewing the long history of the lawsuit, it is impressive how often these individuals turned against one another when the real culprit was the ignorance and apathy of the public and its representatives. Court interventions are one way of shaking up the public and legislative leaders, and one gets the impression that they had some effect in loosening the State's purse strings. But at what price? It is clear from the contributions to this volume that participants will continue to disagree on the price and cost-benefit summation.

Those who really care about improving mental health services in Texas and elsewhere—clients, families, advocates, mental health professionals—have to overcome their differences and constructively agree to disagree on some points, while forging a common agenda and making their case in a more united fashion. The usual divisions between advocates for hospital and community care, adults and children, prevention and treatment, self-help and professional management, have to be confronted and transcended. Mental health interests cannot prevail if advocates waste their energies beating on each other.

There are many challenges ahead. Care for persons with serious mental illness in the community remains uncoordinated and fragmented. Many of the needs of clients for psychiatric services, medical care, appropriate housing, assertive case management, psychosocial rehabilitation and vocational assistance are fully apparent. Persons with mental illness suffer from great stigma and discrimination that extends from daily interactions to questions of insurance and priorities within the overall health care system. If we learn anything from the history of mental health policy in America and elsewhere, it is that advocacy for appropriate care for mental illness must be a continuing endeavor, effectively mobilizing public support and using the mass media and personal contact to keep mental health salient on the public agenda.

Contributors

David Axelrad, M.D., was a psychiatric consultant to the QSO review team. Dr. Axelrad conducts a practice of general psychiatry and pain medicine in Houston, Texas. He is a candidate for certification in psychoanalysis by the Houston/Galveston Institute for Psychoanalysis.

David Bell, Ph.D., was a psychologist at Terrell State Hospital in 1974 when Jenkins v. Cowley was first filed in the federal court. Dr. Bell later served as a mental health consultant to the Court Monitor. He has a practice of psychology in Greenville, Texas.

Hazel Byers was a patient advocate for the QSO review team. She is a member of the Dallas Alliance for the Mentally Ill.

Marilyn Clark, M.A., was a mental health consultant and team leader for the QSO team. She was the Director of Activities Therapy Department at Big Spring State Hospital at the beginning of the process. She currently is Director of the Quality System Oversight Department of Big Spring State Hospital.

Patsy Cheyney was a patient advocate for the Court Monitor. She is member for the San Antonio Alliance for the Mentally Ill and an attorney in San Antonio, Texas.

Cynthia Patton Duran was a client advocate for the Court Monitor. She represented the Texas Mental Health Consumers. She resides in Austin, Texas.

Arthur Farley, M.D., was first a psychiatric consultant to the Court Monitor and then a psychiatric consultant for the QSO team. He is a training psychoanalyst at the Houston/Galveston Institute for Psychoanalysis.

Don A. Gilbert, M.B.A., was superintendent at Terrell State Hospital from 1983 To 1991. He was the Acting Deputy Commissioner for Mental Health Services who designed the QSO Process and negotiated the 1992 Settlement Agreement. He then served as the Executive

Director of the Dallas County MHMR Center. Since 1995 he has served as Commissioner for the Texas Department of Mental Health and Mental Retardation.

Howard H. Goldman, M.D., Ph.D., was a consultant for the Court Monitor on the evaluation of the adequacy of community aftercare. Dr. Goldman is a professor of psychiatry, University of Maryland School of Medicine and is currently Director of Mental Health Policy Studies.

E.R. Hayes, M.D., F.A.C.P., was a consultant to the Court Monitor on internal medicine. He practiced internal medicine in Dallas, Texas.

Genevieve Hearon was a patient advocate for the QSO review team. She is the mother of a schizophrenic daughter, the founder of the Texas Alliance for the Mentally Ill, has served on the Board of Directors of the National Alliance for the Mentally Ill, and she practices advocacy in Austin, Texas.

Douglas Heinrichs, M.D., was a psychiatric consultant to the Court Monitor. He has been a consultant on the use of psychotropic medications for the Maryland Department of Mental Health. He has a practice of general psychiatry in Ellicott City, Maryland.

Lyn Henderson, was a mental health and rights protection consultant for the QSO review team. She is the Rights Protection Officer of Terrell State Hospital

Felicia Korman, M.S.W., was a mental health consultant and team leader for the QSO review team. She is a mental health administrator in Arlington, Texas.

Marty Lumpkin, Ph.D., was a mental health consultant and team leader for the QSO review team. He was the Director of Psychology and then the Director of Program Management at Terrell State Hospital. He has practice of psychology in Terrell, Texas.

Charles McDonald, Ph.D., was a mental health consultant and team leader for the QSO review team and has a practice of psychology in Austin, Texas.

David Mechanic, Ph.D., is the Director of the Institute for Health, Health Care Policy, and Aging Research at Rutgers, the State University of New Jersey, New Brunswick Campus. He is the Rene Dubos University Professor of Behavioral Sciences.

Contributors 285

Susan Medlin was a client advocate for the Court Monitor. She represented the Texas Mental Health Consumers. She continues her advocacy in Austin, Texas.

Gary E. Miller, M.D., was the Commissioner of the Texas Department of Mental Health and Mental Retardation from 1982 through 1988. He had been Deputy Commissioner for Mental Health Services in Texas, Assistant Commissioner of Mental Hygiene in New York, Commissioner of the Georgia Department of Mental Health and Mental Retardation, and Director of Mental Health and Mental Retardation Services for New Hampshire. He currently conducts a practice in general psychiatry in Houston, Texas, and is a Clinical Professor of Psychiatry at the University of Texas Houston Medical School.

David B. Pharis, M.S., M.S.C.R.P., was the Coordinator of the R.A.J. Review Panel from 1981 to 1988 and then the R.A.J. Court Monitor from 1988 to 1997. He currently has a practice of mental health consultation in Austin, Texas.

The Honorable Barefoot Sanders is Senior Judge, U.S. District Court, Northern District of Texas. He presided over R.A.J. v. Gilbert from 1980 to 1997.

Bill Smith, Ph.D., was patient advocate for the QSO review team and represented the Brazos Valley Alliance for the Mentally Ill. He resides in Bryan, Texas.

Anne Younes, Ed.D., worked with Dr. Goldman in the evaluation of the adequacy of community aftercare. She is currently Chief, State Planning and Systems Development Branch, Center for Mental Health Services, Rockville, Maryland.